THE <u>NEW</u> SELF HELP SERIES

COLITIS

Practical advice on these seldom-discussed
complaints, together with a complete
programme for renewed health and vitality.

THE <u>NEW</u> SELF HELP SERIES

COLITIS

ARTHUR WHITE
N.D., D.O.

THORSONS PUBLISHING GROUP
Wellingborough, Northamptonshire

Rochester, Vermont

First published 1987

© THORSONS PUBLISHING GROUP 1987

British Library Cataloguing in Publication Data

White, Arthur
  Colitis: and other bowel disorders. —
  (The New self-help series)
  1. Intestines — Diseases — Treatment
  2. Self-care, Health
  I. Title   II. Series
  616.3'4   RC860

  ISBN 0-7225-1318-6

Printed and bound in Great Britain

Contents

1.

Taboo — Or Not Taboo?

Throughout history, regardless of race, colour or creed, human society has maintained rigid codes of social conduct which have demanded that certain practices and subjects are neither carried out nor discussed openly and publicly.

Many of these taboos had their origins in ancient religious observances, while others grew out of superstitious fears of the retribution which, it was believed, would be visited upon anyone who dared to transgress against the unwritten laws governing social behaviour.

Improved standards of education and communication over the centuries have effectively dispersed many of these irrational fears, while at the same time social inhibitions are being progressively eased or abandoned to an extent that would have appeared inconceivable only a generation or two ago.

Yet today, despite the fact that so-called progressive, liberal thinking has resulted in a degree of freedom of expression which is often embarrassing and even offensive to many people, there is still one subject which is seldom or never discussed socially — namely, the bowel and its functions and malfunctions.

Other organs, such as the heart, the lungs, the stomach, the kidneys, the bladder and even the prostate and genitals are often the subject of open and detailed discussion among even casual acquaintances, whereas the intestines, the colon and the rectum are mentioned, if at all, only in confidential whispers to the closest relatives and friends.

The effect of this exaggerated reticence is that when something goes wrong with this vital component of the digestive system the sufferer is often reluctant to seek professional help and advice. Consequently, a relatively simple functional disorder such as constipation or flatulence goes untreated, or the sufferer resorts to self-medication, relying on traditional family remedies or, more likely, whatever proprietary laxative is being most effectively advertised at the time.

Because, in the natural course of events, relatively minor functional disorders of this kind tend to be self-limiting and self-correcting, the patient's system will eventually resume normal service, and, not unnaturally, credit will be given to the particular remedy which he or she has used.

Again, when faced with a recurrence of the same problem — for reasons which we shall explain later — he or she, naturally, will turn once again to the remedial measures which had apparently proved effective against the earlier attack.

On the face of it, such a course would appear to provide a perfectly logical and satisfactory solution to an embarrassing problem, but there is a serious flaw in such a line of reasoning which, unfortunately, may become apparent only after a lapse of some considerable time — months or even years after the first intestinal hiccup has been forgotten.

That flaw lies in the fact that constipation represents a partial breakdown in the functions of the very complex chain of organs which constitute the digestive system. It is a system which, for all its complexity, is normally extremely efficient and resilient, capable of withstanding the enormous amount and variety of gastronomic abuses to which it is subjected as a result of the radical changes which have taken place, and continue to take place, in regard to present-day feeding habits, and the nature and quality of the products which constitute the modern diet.

It follows, therefore, that signs of failure in any part of such an efficient system will only begin to show themselves after its resources have been under continuing stress for a relatively lengthy period, by which time its very considerable powers of adaptation and tolerance have been strained to the point of exhaustion. At this stage, the overburdened intestine has become so weakened and distended that it is no longer capable of operating efficiently and its vital functions gradually grind to a halt.

Given a reasonably clear understanding of the workings of the body in general and the digestive system in particular, the sufferer would be in a position to analyse the situation objectively and identify possible causes of the functional breakdown and take appropriate corrective action.

Unfortunately, because the inner workings of the bowel are not a socially acceptable subject of discussion, very few people have more than a very hazy conception of what goes on inside the alimentary tract, and so, instead of looking for and removing the *causes* of bowel problems, they resort to the use of laxatives in an attempt to alleviate the *symptoms*.

As a result, a tired and weakened bowel is goaded into some semblance of activity, but because the original causes of its failure have not been removed it is inevitable that the stimulating effect of the laxative will be short-lived. Thus, a vicious circle is established as a result of which the bouts of constipation become progressively more frequent and prolonged.

Eventually, the bowel becomes so distended and congested with a fermenting mass of partially digested food residues that the mucous membranes which line the walls of the intestines and colon become increasingly irritated and inflamed, thus paving the way for the devopment of more serious and chronic disorders such as diverticulitis, appendicitis and colitis.

In succeeding chapters of this book we shall explain in more detail the origins of these very distressing bowel troubles and the reasons why orthodox medical treatment not only fails to provide a solution but actually gives rise to other and often more complex problems.

The human body is such an incredibly complex chemical and physical creation that despite the efforts of the most learned anatomists, physiologists, chemists and many other equally talented scientific workers there is undoubtedly a multitude of secrets which still defy analysis and which will continue to do so well beyond the foreseeable future.

The shelves of our libraries are laden with learned tomes which describe in minute detail the structure of bodily organs, the composition of various tissues and fluids, and the variety of functions which take place within the living body, but the indisputable fact remains that no one has yet succeeded, nor is likely to succeed, in duplicating these various components and assembling them to form a living organism.

Nevertheless, sufficient irrefutable data has been assembled over the years to enable us to understand many of the basic functions of the body and to adduce with reasonable assurance what needs to be done to maintain physical and systemic efficiency; conversely, it is possible, on the basis of that knowledge, to identify those actions and practices which are detrimental to bodily health. Then, by the logical process of harnessing the positive, health-promoting factors and reducing or eliminating those which are physically or nutritionally harmful, we can allow the body to rebuild damaged tissues and restore the normal functional efficiency of its various organs and systems.

It cannot be stressed too strongly that if the maximum and most speedy benefit is to be

obtained from natural treatment it is not
sufficient for the patient to know only what he
or she must do and how to do it; even more
important is a clear understanding of the
reasons *why* certain changes in day-to-day living
style are required and *why* it is advisable to eat
some kind of foods and avoid others.

Only then can he or she appreciate the full
effects of what is being done and the
significance of the gradual changes which are
likely to take place, not only in the specific
symptoms associated with the condition which
is being treated but also their relevance to
physical fitness and bodily health in general.

It is this concern for mutual understanding
between practitioner and patient which is a
fundamental characteristic of the naturopathic
approach in contrast to that of orthodox
medicine.

Largely, though by no means exclusively,
because of intolerable pressure of work, the GP
is rarely able to devote more than a few minutes
to each patient. During this time the doctor will
be able to give only the briefest consideration to
the patient's account of his or her problems and
symptoms, and decide on a possible diagnosis.

The patient will usually leave the consulting-
room with a hastily scribbled prescription for a
pill or potion which, at best, will afford some
degree of comfort or relief, and at worst create
a fresh pattern of symptoms some of which
may well be considerably more troublesome
than those for which treatment was sought in
the first place.

Whether or not the patient will be 'cured' will

depend mainly upon the human body's very considerable capacity for self-repair and self-healing — in spite of, rather than because of, the doctor's intervention.

Because modern medical training and practice are almost exclusively drug-orientated, a patient will receive little or no constructive advice regarding the possible causes of his or her health problems, and with few exceptions doctors tend actively to discourage patients from discussing such matters or asking for guidance as to any steps they may take to guard against a recurrence or worsening of their illness.

It is hardly surprising, therefore, that despite the many millions of pounds that are poured into the National Health Service, the demand for medical, surgical and psychiatric treatment continues to outstrip the available resources, and why heroic measures such as colostomies, gastrectomies and heart, kidney and lung transplants need to be resorted to on an ever-increasing scale.

Such trends will only be reversed when patients are encouraged to take personal responsibility for their own health, which means, in the first place, having a working knowledge of how the various organs and systems of the healthy body function as an integrated unit.

That is why, before discussing the causes and treatment of colitis and other intestinal disorders, it is necessary to clear away the veil of ignorance and mystery concerning the vital role which the bowel plays in the complex physical and chemical processes of digestion and assimilation.

It is a fascinating subject which, once understood, will enable the reader to appreciate that the only real solution to his or her problems lies not in taking laxatives or other palliative medicines but in identifying the causes and removing them.

There is absolutely no valid reason why such a vital component of the digestive system as the bowel should remain shrouded in secrecy in an age when virtually every other bodily organ and function is subjected to the most detailed and intimate examination in the press, and on radio, and television.

So, let us do away with tiresome taboos, so that we can examine the *whole* of the digestive system thoroughly and objectively.

2.

Why Do We Eat?

In reply to the question 'Why do you eat?' it is a
reasonable assumption that most people would
say, 'Because I'm hungry.' Yet it is undoubtedly
true that very few of them would ever have
experienced real hunger, and that the reason
why most of us eat is simply because the clock
says that it is time we had a meal!

Breakfast, lunch and dinner are taken at
predetermined times each day, regardless of
whether there are anything more than the most
superficial indications that food is needed.
Moreover, even the so-called 'hunger pains'
which some people claim to suffer just prior to
mealtimes are all too often habit-induced signals
from a stomach that has become conditioned by
long-established custom to expect the arrival of
food at a specific time each day.

Hunger, according to the *Concise Oxford
Dictionary*, is 'an uneasy sensation, exhausted
condition, caused by want of food'. That is a
fairly accurate definition of *true* hunger — an
indication by the body that its nutritional
reserves are close to exhaustion and that food is

urgently needed to maintain physical activities
and generate body heat.

By strange but perhaps significant contrast,
Black's Medical Dictionary maintains that
'hunger is the term applied to a craving for food
or other substances necessary to body activity.
Hunger for food is *supposed* [our italics] to be
directly produced by strong contractions of the
stomach when it is empty or nearly so.'

A 'craving for food' is by no means
synonymous with 'a need for food'. The
individual who, as a result of habitual
overeating, is grossly overweight and who has
an enormous, bulging abdomen, will often
complain that he is 'always hungry', simply
because his abnormally distended stomach
begins to emit distress signals if it is not
constantly kept filled to capacity.

Again, the spurious hunger-pain tends to
diminish and eventually disappear once the
customary mealtime has passed, even though
no food has been forthcoming, whereas true
hunger pangs and the accompanying weakness
will persist and become increasingly insistent
until the *need* for nourishment has been met.

Between the two extremes there is an
increasingly common type of physiological
hunger which manifests itself as a cry of
distress by a body deprived of vitally essential
nutrients; because, even though food is taken
regularly and in seemingly adequate quantities,
it consists of processed and denatured products
which are seriously deficient, or even totally
devoid, of the vitamins, minerals and other
nutrients which the body needs for tissue

maintenance and growth, and to sustain functional efficiency.

Therefore, if we hark back to the question, 'Why do we eat?' the only logical answer should be: 'To provide the body with the raw materials which are needed to build or restore its many different tissues, to maintain body temperature and to generate sufficient physical and nervous energy to motivate our muscles and organs.'

Until well into the second half of the twentieth century the general public took little or no interest in diet and nutrition, their knowledge of these subjects being confined to the question of whether or not any particular item was 'fattening'. This led to a very widespread preoccupation with the calorie value of various foods, and fortunes have been made by many self-styled experts who jumped on the slimming bandwagon and marketed expensive low-calorie products and special 'crash-diets'.

Sadly, as many disillusioned people found to their cost, the only lasting effect of these gimmicky programmes was to lighten their purses, while any temporary reduction in body weight was rapidly regained once they returned to their 'normal' feeding habits.

The fact is that calorie values are, or should be, of little concern to anyone who seeks to take an intelligent interest in the subject of nutrition and its effect on bodily health. Yet far too many popular health guides still continue to devote a disproportionate amount of space to tables and graphs setting out the daily calorie needs of different types of people according to age, physical characteristics, occupation, etc., while making only the most cursory mention of the other far more important nutritional properties of the foods which constitute the diet of most people today.

Between the wars, the pioneers of natural healing and what was termed 'food reform' were regarded as cranks by the general public, and the nutritional principles which they advocated were ridiculed as 'unscientific' by orthodox doctors and nutritionists, who persisted in maintaining that the type of food we eat has little or no relevance to bodily health and disease.

Perhaps the most glaring of these aberrations was that there was no scientific evidence to support the claims of the 'food cranks' that wholemeal flour and bread were more nutritious than the refined white-flour products. Expert laboratory analysis, they maintained, proved that because most of the important nutrients such as calcium, iron and some of the B vitamins, which are removed from white flour during the milling and refining processes, are required by law to be restored by the subsequent addition of chalk, iron and synthetic vitamins, the claims made on behalf of wholemeal flour and bread by 'health cranks' were not valid.

No account was taken of the subtle *qualitative* differences between the naturally occurring minerals and vitamins in the wholegrain flour and the synthetic products of the chemical laboratory with which white flour is 'fortified'.

Nor was there any appreciation of the vital

role which bran plays in the complex functions of the digestive system. Bran, it was insisted, is an inert and indigestible cellulose which has no nutritional value, and so its removal from flour has no physiological relevance.

On the contrary, it was suggested that foods with a high content of natural fibre could actually be harmful to patients suffering from colitis, diverticulitis and other bowel disorders, who were therefore instructed to omit from their diet such items as fruit, green vegetables and wholegrain cereals. Instead, a bland, non-residue diet was prescribed which included white bread and toast, biscuits, butter, eggs, non-fatty fish, meat extracts, meat jellies and puréed vegetables.

It was well into the second half of the twentieth century before the futility of this advice was appreciated and doctors came to realize that white bread and other refined, low-residue foods were the major causative factor in bowel disorders and that a diet of whole foods with their proper complement of natural fibre is essential not only in maintaining efficient digestive function but also in the treatment of bowel disorders.

This 'discovery' was hailed as a triumph of medical science and an historic breakthrough in the war against disease. The fact that the nature-cure pioneers and food cranks had been advocating such measures for more than half a century was ignored.

Because medical training is almost exclusively drug-orientated, medical students leave their schools and colleges with only the most elementary understanding of the relationship of nutrition to health and disease. They are then pitchforked into a world in which such heavy demands are imposed on them that the average GP's consulting-room resembles a factory conveyor-belt, with a constant succession of patients passing through at intervals of perhaps no more than five or ten minutes.

Under such conditions it would be totally impracticable for doctors to delve into their patient's domestic life in an attempt to discover the causes of the symptoms which they present, and in any case there has been nothing in their training to suggest that such a course of action is in any way desirable or relevant.

The truth is, however, that to a very large degree, *man is what he eats and drinks and breathes*. The extraordinarily complex conglomeration of tissues, fluids, organs and systems which constitute the living human body can only be sustained and motivated by the materials with which it is provided.

In every phase of human endeavour, other than bodily health, it is universally acknowledged that the quality of the end-product is dependent upon the quality of the materials employed in its construction. A first-class machine cannot be built from third-rate metals; good quality furniture cannot be constructed from sub-standard timber; a Rolls Royce car cannot be made from scrap metals and cheap plastics.

All this is self-evident, and yet the vast majority of people today expect their bodies to grow and function efficiently on a diet of processed and denatured materials which are almost entirely devoid of natural nutrients and which, moreover, are coloured, preserved, flavoured and conditioned with a vast range of potentially harmful chemicals.

The primary considerations of food manufacturers today are quick sales, minimum production costs and maximum profits. To achieve these objectives they make liberal use of synthetic substances to bulk out more expensive natural ingredients, then cook it, colour it, flavour it and finally package it in colourful wrappers to ensure maximum eye-appeal and palate appeal in an effort to capture the largest possible share of the market. Millions of pounds are spent on press, television and radio advertising in order to brainwash the consumer into believing that a product is better value for money, tastier and more easily prepared than those of rival manufacturers.

A careful study of the small print on the label will reveal something of the spurious nature of the contents of the pack, provided that the reader can interpret the true meaning of the multi-syllable chemical ingredients or the complex symbols which are supposed to enlighten the customer as to the nature and identity of the various synthetic substances which are used to enhance colour, flavour, etc.

The massive extension of supermarkets and fast-food establishments has brought about a revolution in shopping habits since the middle of the twentieth century, and this has been accompanied by a simultaneous change in the methods used in the production of primary foodstuffs — notably cereal crops and meat.

Intensive farming techniques have long since replaced traditional cultural methods which relied on a large labour force and natural fertilizers. Seed-crop harvests are now boosted artificially with the aid of highly toxic pesticides and chemical growth-stimulants. Free-ranging cattle and pigs are displaced by battery systems in which livestock are kept in crowded pens and cages, deprived of fresh air and exercise, fed on factory-prepared products and treated with hormones to ensure an unnatural growth-rate and to increase milk and egg production.

Because the healthy human body has such a wide-ranging power of adaptability and improvization it could well be argued that, individually, none of these nutritional abuses would give rise to serious harmful effects. Unfortunately, however, there are many people of all ages who cannot be described as really healthy, and their diet consistently contains not one but many dubious products.

When, therefore, they daily consume even small quantities of a multitude of alien chemicals and compound this metabolic abuse by ingesting a mass of refined and denatured products which are seriously deficient in essential vitamins, minerals and fibre it is hardly surprising that sooner or later the overtaxed chemical and functional systems of the body will suffer and break down.

So, having dealt at some length with some of the more common dietetic abuses, let us now look at the other side of the coin and explain briefly the major components of a balanced, health-promoting diet and the metabolic functions which they fulfil.

3.

What Should We Eat?

There is no doubt that Nature acted with the best intentions when she endowed living creatures with the senses of sight, smell and taste which serve the dual purpose of enabling us to select those foods which are wholesome and healthful and reject those which are potentially harmful.

Unfortunately, she did not — and could not — foresee that her most advanced creation, Man, would evolve into a Frankenstein monster which would manipulate and distort the sensory appeal of basic foods to such an extent as to endanger rather than safeguard bodily health.

That is why, in order that we may understand the nutritional causes of ill health, we must first return to basics and explain simply the nature and composition of the foods which constitute a healthful diet and the ingenious processes by which the body extracts and utilizes the essential nutrients which they contain.

For practical purposes, we will confine our review of a very complex subject to the major food components with which many people are already familiar — i.e. carbohydrates, fats, proteins, fibre, vitamins, minerals and water — emphasizing, however, that the order in which these items are listed is more or less inverse to their nutritional and physiological importance.

Carbohydrates are classified mainly as the heat and energy providers in the food chain because of the high-calorie rating of the starches and sugars which are their main components.

Contrary to popular belief, fostered by distorted media representations, carbohydrates are not of themselves responsible for the widespread incidence of obesity in many Western communities. In their natural form and when taken in proper moderation as part of a balanced diet they play a valuable part in many bodily functions; but because of their relatively low cost and the ease with which they can be used to bulk out manufactured products they have tended to displace other far more important foods in the conventional diet. Unfortunately, the carbohydrate which is used for this purpose almost invariably takes the form of 'modified', i.e. refined, starch which is devoid of virtually all nutritional value.

It is only when these denatured foods and other white-flour and white-sugar products such as white bread, cakes, biscuits, polished rice and sweetened breakfast cereals constitute a major part of the daily dietary that obesity and other health problems arise.

It is not widely appreciated that, regardless of whether they are taken in the form of starches or sugars, almost all carbohydrates are transformed first into glucose during the process of digestion and ultimately into fat which is used to generate heat and energy. Once this is understood, it becomes clear why an excess of this dietary component can so readily give rise to obesity, since any surplus that is not required to meet the body's immediate needs is stored away in the tissues and kept in reserve for future use.

A major tenet of balanced natural dietetics is that carbohydrates should constitute not more than 20 per cent of the daily food intake, together with 20 per cent proteins and 60 per cent of the vitamin and mineral-rich fruits, vegetables and salads. Moreover, it is stipulated that this 20 per cent should consist almost exclusively of wholegrain cereal foods in the form of wholewheat bread and crispbread, muesli, unpolished rice, etc.

Sugar as such should have no place in a health-promoting dietary, because it is devoid of all nutrients other than pure sucrose. Thus, it fulfils no physiological function which cannot be performed far more effectively and safely by other foods.

It needs little thought to appreciate the fact that pure sucrose is virtually non-existent in natural foods, and it is only through very sophisticated processes of extraction, refinement and concentration that such a product has become available to man. As a result, it has been estimated that during the last hundred years the consumption of sugar in the UK has increased more than six-fold, with dire consequences in terms of dental decay, obesity, diabetes and coronary heart disease.

Fats: If, as seems to have been proved beyond reasonable doubt, an excess of dietary fats is yet another major causative factor in degenerative diseases of the heart and arteries, it is not surprising that the incidence of these potentially lethal conditions has escalated to such an enormous extent in recent years.

The rapidly increasing trend away from home-cooking in favour of commercially prepared instant dishes, tinned and packeted products and 'take-away' meals has resulted not only in the virtual extinction of vitamins and other nutrients of which fresh, whole foods are the major source, but at the same time the natural nutritional balance of the nation's food has been changed out of all recognition.

Like sugar, fat is a nutrient which seldom constitutes more than a very small component of a whole food, and yet many of the items which comprise the conventional Western diet contain a very high proportion of fat. Fish and chips — said to be one of the most popular dishes in the UK — is a classic example, since fried cod and fried plaice have a fat content of 10 per cent and 14 per cent respectively, and for chipped potatoes the figure is 9 per cent.

Other popular items which have a high level of fat are pork sausages (24 per cent), pork chop (50 per cent), roast pork (40 per cent), fried mutton chop (60 per cent), boiled ham (40 per cent) roast beef (24 per cent), fried bacon (50 per cent), Cheddar cheese (34 per cent), and fried egg (20 per cent). Potato crisps, so dear to the heart and palate of the modern schoolchild, have a fat content of 38 per cent and mixed sweet biscuits have a surprising 31 per cent.

Rather less predictably, perhaps, we find a similarly high-fat content in such diverse products as steamed pudding (20 per cent), shortbread (27 per cent), flaky pastry (42 per cent), eccles cakes (32 per cent), milk chocolate (38 per cent), digestive biscuits (20 per cent) and cream crackers (33 per cent). To top up the fat ration there is of course either butter or margarine — both 85 per cent — spread liberally on bread or biscuits.

Clearly, we do not need to resort to the computer to confirm that vast numbers of people today are assailing their digestive systems with a far greater amount of fat than it was designed to assimilate and utilize, and the resultant problems are compounded by the fact that much of the fat which is consumed is of the 'saturated' variety which is generally believed to be largely responsible for the high incidence of coronary disease.

This, however, is a controversial and extremely complex subject which we need not discuss in detail. Suffice it to say that the allegedly more harmful saturated fats are mainly those of animal origin, i.e. meat and dairy produce, which remain solid at ordinary room temperatures, while the less harmful unsaturated fats are mostly vegetable derivatives which are more likely to be in liquid form.

Whether a fat is more or less harmful is immaterial in the context of balanced feeding, the guiding principle being that the body's requirement of this nutrient will be met adequately by the fat contained, in the correct natural proportions, in the simple whole foods which constitute a balanced, healthful diet.

Proteins are the nutritive materials which are utilized by the body in the vital processes of tissue growth, repair and maintenance and, as is the case with other nutrients, the physiological needs of individuals can vary widely according to such factors as age, physique, energy output, climate, etc.

Nevertheless, a varied diet of whole foods conforming basically to the 60:20:20 formula mentioned earlier in this chapter should serve as a satisfactory nutritional basis except in very exceptional cases.

Generally speaking, the protein foods are considered to comprise all kinds of meat, fish, poultry, eggs, cheese, milk, beans, lentils, peas and certain other pulses, as well as most nuts. Cereals and some vegetables also make a small but none the less useful contribution towards the body's protein needs.

Just as some ill-informed people delude themselves into thinking that, because carbohydrates have a high-calorie content, the more they eat the more energetic they will become, so there is a myth in some quarters that, because protein is the tissue-builder, consuming large quantities of steak and other flesh foods will produce greater strength and increased physical development.

The fallacy of these beliefs cannot be emphasized too strongly, as will be made clear later when we explain the workings of the digestive and assimilative systems. At this stage, however, it may be timely to liken the processes by which the body's tissues are maintained to those which are employed by a housewife when she bakes a loaf. She knows that good quality, fresh ingredients must be used in carefully measured quantities, and that any deviation from the recipe will almost inevitably result in a disappointing end-result when the bread finally emerges from the oven.

If so much care is needed when carrying out such a simple task as baking a loaf, it is not difficult to appreciate the far greater need to ensure that the immensely complex human organism is provided with only the highest quality materials in the right quantities and proportions if it is to develop and function efficiently.

This is a lesson which simply *must* be learned and acted upon if health is to be restored and maintained.

Fibre achieved cult status when the medical establishment belatedly — and reluctantly — accepted the fact that 'roughage' is not simply an inert and indigestible component of vegetables, cereals and fruit which passes through the human digestive system and is excreted without serving any useful physiological function.

As we have mentioned already, in Chapter 2, the nature-cure pioneers were denouncing refined carbohydrates — white flour, polished rice, white sugar, etc. — as a major causative factor in constipation, colitis, diverticulitis and other common digestive disorders for more than half a century before this seemingly self-evident fact was 'discovered' by the medical profession.

Then, as is so often the case when a 'medical breakthrough' is proclaimed, commercial interests leapt on to a potentially profitable bandwagon and the shelves of the supermarket and chemists shops were soon piled high with 'high-fibre' food products.

Sadly, 'moderation' is a word which has no place in the vocabulary of the advertising and marketing professions, who used their skills to such good effect that a gullible public was quickly persuaded that 'you cannot have too much of a good thing', whether it be vitamins, minerals, proteins — or fibre.

Here again logical reasoning *must* provide the yardstick when judging the validity of any such commercially motivated nutritional claim. For example, if we remember that bran constitutes only 13 per cent of the total wheatgrain we can appreciate that if two average slices of wholewheat bread, weighing 60g, are eaten the digestive system will be dealing with slightly less than 8g of bran, the remaining 52g being made up of a balanced mixture of starch, protein, fat and water.

If, however, two tablespoons of bran are taken in addition to the same or a greater amount of bread, as may be the effect of following a 'high-fibre diet', a totally different problem is imposed on the alimentary canal in the form of a mass of bulky and mostly indigestible roughage which could well impose an intolerable burden on a digestive system which is unaccustomed to dealing with even a modest amount of any such material.

This is why many of those who are persuaded to adopt a high-fibre diet in an attempt to relieve constipation, colitis, etc. find that any apparent benefit is short-lived, and they are then plagued with flatulence and abdominal distension.

Clearly, the logical, natural approach is to 'make haste slowly' by adopting a simple but balanced diet of whole foods in which *all* nutrients are combined in their proper quantities and proportions, so as to rebuild and re-educate the weakened digestive and assimilative organs, and encourage them to function naturally and efficiently.

A tenet of natural healing which cannot be stressed too strongly or too frequently is: No matter what one's health problem may be, the only safe and logical course is one that is based on simplicity and moderation. Extremes invariably result in complications in the long run, whether they take the form of supplementation, extraction or concentration.

Vitamins: According to *Black's Medical Dictionary*, vitamins are:

> ... a group of substances which exist in minute quantities in natural foods, and which are necessary to normal nutrition, especially in connection with growth and development. Several of them have now been synthesized. When they are absent from the food, defective growth takes place in young animals and children, and in adults various diseases arise... Persistent deprivation of one or other vitamin is apt to lead to a state of lowered health.

The term 'vitamin' is of course derived from the word 'vital' — meaning essential to life — and we would stress the fact that, as stated in the dictionary definition, the various vitamins exist *only in natural foods*. Therefore, to suggest that there can be such a thing as a 'synthetic' vitamin is a contradiction in terms, inasmuch as nothing produced by a chemist in a laboratory can possibly duplicate exactly the original substance formulated by Nature as part of a living — *vital* — plant organism. Nor, when it is consumed, will it have the same metabolic effect, not merely because of incomprehensible differences in its chemical structure, but, even more importantly, because it will not be compounded with other nutrients in the precise proportions and combinations which distinguish a natural whole food from the man-made — and man *un*-made — conglomeration of bits and pieces to be found on the shelves of supermarkets.

One of the first lessons which many of us were taught in the school chemistry class emphasized the need for the utmost care when mixing chemical compounds, because even a slight deviation from the specified formula could have very serious consequences. How, then, can we expect such a complex chemical organism as the human body to function if it is fuelled with a hotch-potch of cooked and processed rubbish, stripped of many natural nutrients and then 'fortified' with synthetic chemical substitutes?

Although vitamins play such an important part in bodily functions they are needed only in the most minute quantities. Many of them, indeed, seem to serve merely as catalysts, which means that they do not themselves undergo a chemical reaction when ingested but, by their very presence, they can determine the speed and extent to which other chemical substances react with each other when they are brought together.

Thus, just one twenty-thousandth of an ounce of vitamin B_1 is all that the average person needs to obtain from his daily food ration; but in some parts of the world where polished rice or white flour forms the staple diet, the inhabitants are susceptible to beri-beri — a severe nerve disease — because the cereal husk which carries almost all of this vitamin is removed in the course of the refining process. Beri-beri was in fact the first vitamin deficiency disease to be specifically identified, and the discovery was made when a population changed from a diet which consisted almost exclusively of brown rice to one in which polished white rice predominated.

Scurvy is another and even better-known vitamin-deficiency disease which, for hundreds of years, plagued the early mariners who pioneered the sea routes around the world. Captain Cook is credited with having been the first to realize that the dreaded disease could be prevented during a long sea voyage by ensuring that his crew were provided with fresh vegetables and fruit, including oranges and lemons, at every opportunity when he circumnavigated the globe and explored

Australia and New Zealand in the latter years of the eighteenth century.

Some twenty years earlier, however, a Scots naval surgeon had published a treatise in which he described a series of trials which showed that scurvy could be both cured and prevented by hygienic measures combined with an adequate dietary which included fresh oranges and lemons. Such is the conservatism of the establishment, however, that it was not until forty years after this treatise was published that the British Admiralty was persuaded to put these precepts into practice. As a result, scurvy was almost immediately banished from the Royal Navy, which was to prove of inestimable value in the subsequent Napoleonic campaigns.

At that time, of course, the existence of vitamins was not even suspected, and another century passed before it was found that vitamin C, in the form of ascorbic acid, was the active principle in fresh fruit and vegetables which prevented scurvy.

There is still considerable controversy as to the number and nature of those vitamins which so far are believed to have been identified, but there is no doubt that far more remains to be discovered than is already known about these complex nutrients.

What is more, there is an equally wide division of opinion concerning the recommended daily allowances (RDAs) which 'experts' in various countries believe to be necessary to maintain health in various age-groups.

Clearly, then, it would be futile for us to make

any attempt to modify or control our daily vitamin intake or to try to assess whether any symptom of ill health is attributable to a deficiency or excess of any specific nutrient, quite apart from the fact that the body's need of vitamins will vary widely from day to day.

We will return to this problem later and offer what we consider to be the only logical solution to the perplexing problem of providing a balanced and adequate dietary.

Minerals: Complex as is the part played by vitamins in the chemistry of the human body, there is little doubt that the role of minerals in our metabolic processes presents even greater problems for the physiologist.

For many decades, clinical and laboratory experiments of almost unbelievable complexity have been conducted by research scientists; but time after time their findings have been subsequently challenged or disproved when it has been found that the introduction into the experimental programme of a hitherto unsuspected factor brought about a vastly different reaction within the tissues and organs of the subject of the study.

This is not surprising when it is remembered that no two individuals have precisely the same physical structure, that there are wide variations in the functional efficiency of their organs and vital systems and, indeed, that all of these factors change constantly in each person from day to day, month to month, season to season and year to year throughout life.

Therefore, although we can safely accept the fact that certain minerals such as iron, calcium, magnesium, phosphorus, etc. are essential to the health and structural integrity of the human body, any assertions as to the precise quantities and combinations needed must be regarded with the utmost scepticism and suspicion. No matter how impressive are the academic qualifications of the 'experts' who make such assertions, it is certain that there are undreamed of complications still to be elucidated which sooner or later will change fundamentally the significance and validity of their findings.

The extent to which even the most highly esteemed nutritionists can draw wrong conclusions on the basis of meticulous and seemingly logical experimental findings is exemplified by the classic example of the effect of phytic acid on the nutritional properties of wholewheat bread.

In 1925 Sir Edward Mellanby found that puppies reared on a diet containing little calcium and vitamin D, but a large amount of bread, grew rapidly but developed severe rickets. Further experiments showed that the deformities were more severe in the animals fed on oatmeal than in those given wholewheat flour, and least severe in those fed on white flour.

Subsequent experiments revealed that the severity of the rickets was directly proportional to the phytic acid content of the flour and, not unnaturally, the experts concluded that the body's calcium needs were more readily satisfied by white flour than by wholemeal, which had a higher phytic acid content.

Consequently, when, during the early stages of the 1939–1945 war, it became necessary to conserve grain supplies by replacing white bread with a 'national loaf' containing more of the whole grain, the Government was persuaded by its medical advisers to add calcium carbonate (chalk) to the flour in order to counteract the supposed effect of the higher phytic acid content.

It was some years later, after the end of the war, that doubts concerning the validity of the earlier research began to arise. On closer examination of the original findings it seemed logical to ask why — if phytic acid was the cause of rickets in puppies fed on wholewheat flour — was the disease not prevalent in those people living in parts of Scotland where porridge — made from oats which have a higher phytic acid content than wholewheat flour — is a staple part of the diet?

The answer, apparently, is that the ever-adaptable human digestive system has developed an enzyme which neutralizes the phytic acid so that the calcium in wholegrain cereals is readily available for the maintenance of the bones and teeth.

It is, of course, likely that this is an oversimplification of a complex metabolic conundrum, but the fact remains that brilliant nutritionists remained blind to the fact that in vast populations throughout the world rickets is virtually unknown, despite the fact that they depend on a diet containing a preponderance of wholegrain cereals.

Today, many decades later, the false view

that white flour is a better source of calcium than wholewheat is still promulgated in some quarters by commercial milling interests.

The lesson to be drawn from this simple case-history is that, for the layman at least, logical reasoning is a far more reliable guide than scientific laboratory experiments when attempting to assess the body's nutritional needs — whether they be vitamins, minerals, fatty acids, or any of the multitude of substances which constitute a wholesome, balanced diet.

Surely, also, it is logical to assume that a diet of simple whole foods in their natural form is more likely to provide the body with the raw materials needed for growth, repair and maintenance than a commercially processed and denatured product which has been fortified, texturized, coloured, preserved, flavoured, stabilized, emulsified and bulked or concentrated to such an extent that the end-product owes far more to the chemical laboratory than it does to the farmer and his fellow food-producers.

Water: Very few people appreciate the vitally important role which water fulfils in regard to the functional efficiency of their bodies, and it is probable that even fewer consider the effect on their digestive and metabolic systems of the various liquids which they imbibe so freely throughout their lives.

Yet it is undoubtedly true to say that the nature and quality of the beverages which we drink are just as important, if not more so, as those of the foods which we eat.

The body of an average man weighing 65kg

(10 st) contains no less than 40 litres (9 gal) of water, 60 per cent of which is bound up within the cells which form our various tissues and organs. The remaining 40 per cent is made up of the fluids which circulate around the body carrying nutrients to the tissues, removing waste products, and facilitating the vast range of chemical processes which make life possible.

Just as real hunger is seldom experienced by the vast majority of people living in the industrialized nations of the West, so true thirst is an equally rare phenomenon for most of us. We tend to drink much as we eat — not because of physiological need but according to the dictates of custom and the clock, and little or no thought is given to the nature and composition of our beverages or the effects they are likely to have once they have passed our lips.

It has been estimated that the daily fluid intake of a man leading a mainly sedentary life will total approximately 2.6 litres ($4\frac{1}{2}$ pt), nearly 90 per cent of which is derived directly from beverages and the water-content of our foods, the remainder being the product of complex chemical reactions which take place when starches, proteins and fats are digested.

During the same period an almost identical quantity of fluid is excreted — 50 per cent being voided as urine via the kidneys, 2 per cent in the faeces via the bowel, and the remaining 40 per cent being lost in the form of vapour from the lungs and perspiration from the skin.

Although it is self-evident that thirst would be quenched naturally by simply drinking fresh spring water, it is probably true to say that, among urban communities, only very few people ever drink water in its natural state. Instead, they have become habituated from childhood to taking frequent cups of tea, coffee, cocoa or milk or quantities of beer, spirits, 'squashes' or other much-publicized commercial concoctions.

While it is true that modern tap water has little in common with natural spring water, it is certainly an infinitely more healthful beverage than any of the alternatives mentioned above. These contain chemical substances which are at best alien in terms of human nutrition and at worst potentially harmful to one or more of the organs which are responsible for such vital functions as extracting essential nutrients from our foods and drinks, and filtering out and excreting poisonous or unwanted substances.

It is, of course, the digestive tract, the kidneys and the liver which are mainly responsible for these functions and which, therefore, are most at risk from the gastronomic abuses which are unthinkingly imposed upon them by so many people. The qualitative deficiencies with which these organs have to cope are often compounded by quantitative excesses, since most people today tend to drink to excess, sometimes in the mistaken belief that it is desirable to 'flush out the kidneys' from time to time in much the same way as they would flush out the sink. They fail to appreciate that the kidneys are not merely a drain but are an extremely delicate filtering system and are also responsible for maintaining the body's very finely poised fluid balance and carrying out many highly specialized chemical procedures.

Any unnecessary work-load that is imposed on them, therefore, must inevitably impair their efficiency and lead eventually to weakness and possible breakdown. There is little doubt that the massive increase in the chemical contamination of commerical food products and beverages has been a major factor in the escalation in the incidence of kidney disease, particularly in children and young adults.

Where drinks are concerned, therefore, the guiding principle for anyone who has any concern for bodily health is to drink only sufficient to satisfy natural thirst and to rely mainly on water or natural fruit or vegetable juices diluted with 50 per cent water.

It will be readily appreciated that since the water content of our food meets approximately 40 per cent of the body's fluid requirement, the need for other liquid refreshment will be substantially reduced if the diet contains a high proportion of fruit and vegetables, which have a very high water content, and proportionately fewer cereal and protein foods which contain substantially less fluid.

If any reader of the foregoing is wondering why it is thought necessary to devote so much attention to the basic dietary components we would remind him or her that colitis and other bowel diseases are not localized disorders but are indicative of a fundamental breakdown of the body's ability to maintain vital organic functions. Bearing in mind what we have said already concerning the tremendous capacity of living organisms to tolerate abuse and misuse, it will be appreciated that any such breakdown will occur only when the safeguarding mechanisms have been strained beyond endurance.

Therefore, if any attempt to repair damaged tissue and restore normal functions is to have any hope of success the sufferer *must* first understand the role of proper nutrition in providing the raw materials needed to make good damage which, no doubt unwittingly, has been inflicted on the digestive system in general and the intestines in particular.

Having, it is hoped, achieved this, there remains one further physiological mystery to be elucidated before we can consider more specifically the nature and causes of the various bowel disorders and the natural treatment measures which alone can provide a lasting solution to these distressing problems.

In the next chapter, therefore, we shall conduct the reader on a tour through the length of the alimentary canal, explaining as we go what happens to the food we eat and some of the chemical processes to which it is subjected in order that the various nutritive components may be extracted and utilized.

4.

The Miracle of Digestion

From the time food is taken into the mouth until the unwanted residues are excreted from the rectum it will have travelled some 8m (30 ft) along a basically tubular system — the alimentary canal (see Fig. 1, page 47) and been subjected to an amazing variety of physical and chemical processes.

Indeed, the first phase of digestion actually commences *before* any food enters the mouth, because the mere sight and smell of food triggers off the secretion of saliva from three pairs of glands strategically placed around the throat and under the tongue. Thus, when we commence to eat the process of mastication will break down the food which is then mixed with the saliva into a semi-liquid mass which can pass easily into the oesophagus ready for its long journey down the alimentary canal — a journey which may take twenty-four hours or more to complete.

Having descended through the chest cavity the oesophagus passes through the thick, muscular diaphragm and into the abdomen, carrying the semi-liquid food mass into the stomach. Already, however, any starchy components of the meal will have been partially digested by exposure to enzymes in the saliva, which is why the importance of thorough mastication needs to be emphasized.

Propelled by alternating waves of contraction and relaxation, known as peristalsis, the food enters the stomach, the muscular walls of which subject it to a slow, churning process in order to mix it with various digestive juices, including hydrochloric acid, which are secreted by millions of tiny glands situated in the stomach walls. The latter, incidentally, are protected from the erosive effect of the acid by mucous secretions.

A series of complex chemical processes then takes place which begins the breakdown of the protein elements of the meal, while allowing the digestion of the carbohydrates to continue. This stage of digestion may last for four or five hours until eventually a valve at the base of the stomach will open, allowing the partially digested liquid, known as chyme, to pass on into the duodenum, which is the first part of the small intestine.

It is in the duodenum, which is approximately 30cm (12 in) in length, that the next stage of digestion begins, for it is here that two further secretions, bile and pancreatic juice, are released into the intestine. Bile is a thick, bitter liquid which is formed in the liver and is then stored in the gall-bladder, from which it is discharged into the duodenum through a narrow tube — the bile-duct. Its main function is to emulsify the fatty constituents of foods, in which action it is complemented by secretions from the pancreas. The latter organ also releases four powerful ferments which respectively play a further important role in the digestion of fats, milk, proteins and starches during the passage of the chyme through the jejunum and into the small intestine — a convoluted muscular tube measuring some 5 metres (16 ft) in all.

It is only at this stage that the absorption of the end-products of the digestive processes commences, the breakdown of the food into its nutritive components having been finally completed by enzymes secreted by the intestine and bacteria which are normal inhabitants of a healthy bowel. Their main role is to complete the decomposition and fermentation of proteins and carbohydrates and to manufacture some of the B vitamins.

Incidentally, alcohol is the only substance which is absorbed into the blood-stream directly through the tissues of the stomach lining, which is why breath-testing provides a speedy and relatively reliable means of confirming drunkenness.

Water passes very quickly from the stomach into the intestines and much of it is extracted into the circulatory system within a very few minutes.

The main bulk of the semi-solid chyme, however, is further liquefied into a creamy fluid, chyle, which then begins a lengthy passage through the small intestine. This process may occupy a period of several hours, during which

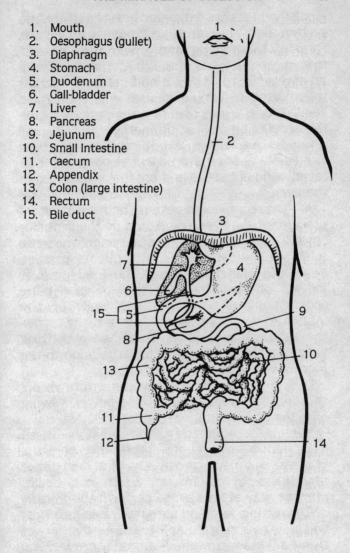

1. Mouth
2. Oesophagus (gullet)
3. Diaphragm
4. Stomach
5. Duodenum
6. Gall-bladder
7. Liver
8. Pancreas
9. Jejunum
10. Small Intestine
11. Caecum
12. Appendix
13. Colon (large intestine)
14. Rectum
15. Bile duct

Figure 1   Diagram of the Alimentary Canal.

emulsified fats are extracted into the lymphatic system and the remaining nutrients, in the form of salts, sugar and amino acids derived from proteins, pass through the walls of the intestine into the blood-stream to be transported to various tissues where they are needed for the purposes of growth or repair, or the production of heat or energy.

Any excess which is not required to meet immediate needs is stored by the body either as fat in various tissues and organs or as sugar in the liver.

All the complex digestive and assimilative processes have been completed by the time the chyle leaves the small intestine and enters the colon via the caecum. Throughout its passage down the alimentary canal the food mass is moved onward by a series of peristaltic contractions of the muscular walls of the intestines — a process which eventually carries the indigestible residues, combined with toxic waste materials, through the large colon to the rectum where is awaits excretion.

During the latter stage, water is drawn off through the walls of the large bowel, leaving only the semi-solid faecal mass.

It must be emphasized that what has been described in this chapter represents only the briefest summary of the chemical and other procedures by means of which our bodies manage, day after day, to perform the miracle of converting fats and carbohydrates into heat and energy, and proteins into the vast variety of tissue substances needed for bodily growth and maintenance.

However, even this brief outline will, it is hoped, enable the reader to appreciate the vital importance of restoring impaired digestive and assimilative organs to full functional efficiency, and to recognize the role which proper nutrition must play if this desirable aim is to be realized.

Moreover, it provides a working knowledge of the various organs which comprise the alimentary canal, which is essential if we are to understand the course of events which has caused the various bowel defects and abnormalities which plague so many people today.

5.

What Has Gone Wrong?

In the preceding chapters we have explained why we eat, what we should eat, and what happens to our food once it has been consumed. It is now time for the reader to utilize this knowledge and to examine his or her own diet and habits of living generally in order to understand what has caused a breakdown in the chain of organs and systems which comprise the alimentary canal.

From what has been said already the reader will almost certainly have more than a suspicion that the traditional diet and eating habits are the front runners when it comes to apportioning responsibility for colitis, diverticulitis, appendicitis, flatulence, 'irritable bowel syndrome' and, indeed, most other digestive and bowel disorders.

With even a sketchy knowledge of how the digestive system functions and how food is utilized by the body, it must be patently clear that most of the packeted, tinned and bottled products which are piled into the supermarket trolleys are not only grossly deficient in regard to nutritional properties but are also laced liberally with preservatives, colourings, flavourings and other products of the laboratory which constitute a chemical cocktail which cannot fail to play havoc with the delicately balanced metabolism of the human body.

There is, of course, no such thing as an 'average' human being, nor can there be an 'average' diet, but it is likely that the basic meal pattern for many people today would conform fairly closely to the following regime.

Pride of place at breakfast time would almost certainly be taken by one of the many packeted cereals made from flaked wheat, oats or corn, cooked with salt and sugar, flavoured and 'fortified' with various synthetic vitamins and minerals such as iron, calcium, etc. These will be served usually with milk and more sugar.

To supplement this dish, or as an alternative, there may be white bread or toast and marmalade, or beans on toast, or spaghetti on toast, or for a 'big eater' a fried egg or two with bacon, or sausage, and perhaps fried bread. A cup or two of tea or coffee will round off the meal.

The main meal of the day will almost certainly consist of meat in one form or another, possibly sausages or a hamburger, or fried fish, with chips or boiled potatoes and perhaps boiled carrots, cabbage or peas. This is likely to be followed by some kind of pudding or pastry with custard, or sweetened stewed or tinned fruit, or an 'instant dessert mix' concocted of such exotic ingredients as modified starch, sugar, whey powder, hydrogenated vegetable oil, emulsifiers, gelling agents, casseinate, lactose, flavourings, salt, colouring and antioxidant!

The nature of the third meal of the day probably varies more than the others depending upon business or domestic commitments, but for many people it may consist of sandwiches of white bread filled with cheese, meat or tinned fish; or cold meat or an egg with white bread or toast, followed perhaps by white bread and jam or a cake or pastry.

These meals also will be washed down with at least two cups of tea or coffee or a glass of beer, and more tea or coffee will probably be taken during the morning and afternoon breaks.

Such a dietary plan is conspicuously lacking in fresh fruit and salads, and it is likely that any cooked vegetables or fruits will have been carefully peeled, thus depriving them of much of their natural roughage. In addition, bread and cereals will almost certainly have been made from refined white flour from which the bran will have been removed during the milling process.

Clearly, then, such a diet will have lost a considerable proportion of its original nutrient value, the detrimental effects of which on the biochemical balance of the body will have been further increased by any extraneous chemicals which have been added to the food by commercial processors.

Anyone with the most elementary knowledge of chemistry will know that even slight variations of errors in a chemical formula will almost certainly have disastrous effects on the outcome of any laboratory process, and although the human organism has a very considerable capacity for adaptation and selection, it is inevitable that such a complex and delicately balanced chemical entity will suffer and eventually break down under the type of abuse to which it is so frequently subjected.

To further compound these qualitative problems we have to recognize the fact that overeating and indulgence in excessively bulky meals is widespread today, as is evident by the fact that obesity is such a major cause of concern.

As was explained in the preceding chapter, during the final stages of digestion nutrients are taken up by the blood-stream and carried to various parts of the body, but any that are surplus to immediate requirements are stored away in the form of fat or sugar, thus affording a strategic reserve to be drawn on to meet any subsequent food shortage. Because of the almost universal habit of eating adequate meals at regular intervals throughout the day such emergencies rarely if ever arise, and so the fatty reserves continue to accumulate to the point where they become both a physical and metabolic burden on the individual.

Meanwhile, the sheer bulk of food that is consumed poses very considerable problems for the alimentary canal. A 'normal' stomach has a total capacity of approximately $1\frac{1}{2}$ litres ($2\frac{1}{2}$ pt) and so it is quite capable of accommodating quite a large meal, although it would come under some strain if, say, a pint of beer or two cups of tea or coffee were to be taken at the same time.

We know, however, that this mass of food and liquid — including the various digestive juices — will remain in the stomach for four or five hours, during which time it will be churned slowly and rhythmically by muscular contractions to ensure thorough mixing. It requires little imagination to appreciate the fact that a fully distended stomach will perform these functions far less efficiently than one that is only lightly laden.

In the first place, a fully stretched muscle is much less efficient than one that is working well within its normal capacity and, at the same time, a tightly packed mass of food cannot be turned and kneaded with anything like the same facility as could a smaller quantity.

Moreover, the normal quantity of gastric juices and hydrochloric acid will be required to combine with an excessive amount of food material, thus inevitably the subsequent digestive processes will be performed less efficiently and completely.

It is likely that in order to relieve the strain imposed upon it an overladen stomach will pass some of the partially digested food prematurely into the duodenum, thus imposing problems on the intestines, liver and gall-bladder. Finally, the conventional meal is virtually devoid of natural fibre, the presence of which is known to trigger off the peristaltic contractions which propel the unwanted food residues into and along the colon to the rectum. As a consequence there is a gradual build-up in the large bowel which becomes increasingly distended. At the same time fluid continues to be drawn off through the walls of the colon so that the faecal mass becomes hard and evacuation more difficult.

Clearly, then, an excessive consumption of denatured and badly balanced food material is the key factor which is primarily responsible for the onset of constipation, thus paving the way for more serious bowel problems, but the harmful effects of such a diet do not end there. Persistent indigestion and constipation invariably have a very debilitating effect on the sufferer, leading to a feeling of lethargy and reluctance to engage in even moderately strenuous activities, particularly in the case of those who are also overweight. Moreover, many people today lead sedentary lives, relying on a car or public transport services and the radio or television for entertainment instead of walking or taking part in active recreational or sporting activities. As a result, their muscles become weak, their breathing shallow and the efficiency of the heart and circulation is impaired.

The health implications of these defects are far more serious than many people appreciate. Obvious signs of bodily deterioration are the increasing distension of the abdomen, shortness of breath and a tendency to feel the cold in winter and to perspire excessively in summer. In many cases postural changes become steadily more pronounced, e.g. rounded shoulders, hollowed back and sunken chest.

Less obvious, but potentially more serious, are the insidious degenerative changes in vital organs such as the heart, arteries and liver, all of which depend directly or indirectly on muscular activity for their functional efficiency.

It is a basic law of nature that the development of muscle tissue is directly proportional to the amount of work that it is called upon to perform. Anyone who has been confined to bed for a week or two will have experienced the feeling of weakness that results from even a short spell of inactivity, and the rapid recovery of strength that ensues once normal activities are resumed.

Athletes, of course, are fully aware of this phenomenon and their training schedules are carefully graduated with a view to increasing the severity and duration of those activities which are known to develop the muscular systems which are specifically involved in the performance of their chosen speciality.

The heart is a muscular organ which collects oxygenated blood from the lungs and pumps it along the network of arteries to every part of the body. Having delivered oxygen and nutrients and collected waste products, the blood begins its return journey through the veins to the heart, but for this purpose the pumping effect of the heart is no longer operative. Instead, the body relies largely on the alternating contraction and relaxation of the muscles around the veins to force the blood upward, against the pull of gravity, aided by an ingenious system of valves which prevent any reflux movement of the blood when muscular pressure is relaxed.

Thus, an activity such as walking, which necessitates rhythmic movements of the legs and arms, not only facilitates the circulation in those limbs but also initiates deep-breathing which, by expanding and contracting the lungs and raising and lowering the muscular diaphragm, sucks blood up through the abdomen into the chest cavity and so back to the heart.

Few people are aware that blood is not the only fluid which circulates throughout the body. A separate system of vessels, similar to blood corpuscles and veins, collects another vital fluid — lymph — which is derived from the blood and which plays an equally important role in the healing of wounds, removal of tissue wastes, destruction of harmful bacteria, and the elimination of dirt and other foreign matter which may have gained access to the tissues, e.g. through a wound or other injury.

Lymph, which is a clear watery fluid similar to blood plasma, exudes from the blood capillaries into the tissues where it deposits nutrient materials and absorbs waste products from the cells. It is then taken up by the capillaries of the lymphatic vessels which gradually unite at various strategic points in the body, notably the groins, the armpits and the neck, where they pass through small, nodular glands. It is here that harmful substances and bacteria are trapped and destroyed, after which the purified lymph flows on up to the neck where it re-enters the blood-stream and is returned to the heart via the large jugular vein.

An understanding of the vital protective functions of the lymphatic system is important because, like the veins, the lymph vessels rely very largely on muscular contractions in order to function efficiently. Regular exercise is therefore doubly important if recovery from illness or functional disorders is to be achieved as quickly and efficiently as possible.

When, as is often the case, lack of regular exercise is coupled with a sedentary occupation, we are faced with yet another problem in our search for the causes of bowel disorders — namely faulty posture. When we sit for long periods in a car, at a desk or workbench, at the meal-table, or in an easy chair in front of the television, the spine is curved, the chest is cramped and the abdomen is constricted, with the result that blood cannot circulate efficiently and the functions of the digestive organs are impaired.

This review of the various factors which play a part in the insidious development of bowel disorders would not be complete without some reference to the effects of stress on the digestive system. Sufferers from colitis, in particular, are often told that their symptoms are caused by 'nerves' and overwork. Such a diagnosis ignores the various dietetic and other errors with which we have dealt already at some length, but there is no doubt that occupational and domestic stresses can and do aggravate, and in some cases perpetuate, certain digestive and bowel disorders.

It is, however, not very helpful to tell a patient that his colitis or duodenal ulcer is caused by nerves unless he is also told *why* this should be so. Only when the connection between causes and symptoms is clearly understood is the patient able to appreciate the nature of his problems and take appropriate corrective action.

In our description of the chemical and physical functions of the digestive system we explained that the passage of food along the alimentary canal triggered the release of various enzymes and the opening and closing of the sphincters (valves) which allow the food to pass on from one part of the system to the next. When, however, an individual is faced with a stressful situation, the body reacts immediately by cutting off energy from the digestive organs and switching all its resources to the heart, lungs and muscles in readiness to deal with whatever threat caused the alarm to be raised.

If the shock is of terrifying proportions the body's reactions will be equally dramatic and any undigested food in the stomach will be vomited immediately and the bowels may be similarly activated. When, however, a person is subjected to a lesser degree of worry or anxiety the digestive processes will be slowed down or temporarily halted, the mouth will remain dry because the secretion of saliva is inhibited, as also will the release into the stomach and intestines of the various digestive juices.

In normal circumstances this suspension of digestive functions will be short-lived, and 'normal services will be resumed' as soon as the stressful situation has passed. When, however, a person is subjected to continuous worry and anxiety either at work or in domestic life, the effect is far more insidious and the end-results more serious inasmuch as his digestive functions are almost constantly impaired. As a consequence, the food he eats will pass very slowly along the alimentary canal, and because the gastric secretions are inhibited it will be only partially digested. Nutrients will not be assimilated and the bulky residues will ferment in the intestines and colon causing distension, congestion and inflammation of the mucous membranes which line these organs.

It is not without significance that colitis is quite common among men in their thirties and forties — the time of life when career pressures and financial commitments are often heavy and when, as a consequence, domestic stress is likely to arise.

These, then, are the major causes of the bowel disorders with which this book is concerned, and the treatment measures which we shall shortly prescribe will all be directed towards eliminating or correcting past errors and allowing the innate curative and reparative powers of the body to operate as efficiently as possible.

It is almost certain, however, that many if not all of those who are seeking help in these pages will have been trying — for many years perhaps — to find relief from their health problems through the medium of pills and medicines, either prescribed by their GPs or purchased from a drug store or supermarket on the strength of the claims made for their wonderful therapeutic properties in press and television advertisements.

Because many of these drugs do not merely fail to afford more than very short-lived temporary relief of the painful and embarrassing symptoms of bowel disorders but actually perpetuate the problems they are supposed to 'cure', our next concern is to explain why this sorry state of affairs is inevitable.

6.

The Facts and the Fallacies

When, in years to come, the history of medicine comes to be rewritten it is likely that the twentieth century will be dubbed 'The Age of the Miracle Drugs', for scarcely a decade has passed without a 'major breakthrough' being claimed by one or other of the giant international pharmaceutical companies.

Insulin, the sulpha drugs, cortisone and the antibiotics are but a few of the discoveries which we were told would bring salvation to suffering humanity and which not only failed to live up to their early promise but were found, sooner or later, to cause such dire side-effects that they are now prescribed only with very considerable circumspection.

It is not just the very sophisticated 'prescription only' drugs that have been indicted in this way. Many of the so-called 'household remedies' were also found to have unexpected harmful effects, as a result of which they have largely fallen into disuse.

There is no doubt that some of the latter have

played a contributory role in the early history of the bowel disorders with which we are concerned. At one time, for example, it was routine for parents to dose their children with ferrous suphate whenever they appeared to be pale and lackadaisical on the assumption that they were anaemic and needed an iron tonic. It was found subsequently that, not surprisingly, iron in this form is not metabolized by the body in the same way as the natural mineral in foods, and that even in normal therapeutic doses it could have irritant and corrosive effects on the mucous membranes lining the alimentary canal, causing pain, constipation, diarrhoea and vomiting in approximately 15 per cent of patients treated.

Larger doses were of course even more destructive of the bowel tissues to the extent of causing stricture and circulatory failure and, in some cases, severe haemorrhage, convulsions, coma and even death due to liver failure.

Aspirin is another drug which was promoted as a safe and effective remedy for virtually all common ailments from colds and headaches to fevers and rheumatoid arthritis. Over the years countless millions of tablets have been sold freely over the counters of chemists and supermarkets, and it was not until relatively high doses of the drug were prescribed for the relief of arthritic pain that the hitherto unsuspected side-effects began to reveal themselves. They include dizziness, tinnitus, sweating, nausea, vomiting and mental confusion.

To quote from one of the foremost

pharmaceutical reference books which devotes more than four closely printed pages to these harmful effects, their treatment and the precautions to be observed when prescribing the drug:

> An important toxic effect which may occur even with small doses (of aspirin) is irritation of the gastric mucosa and resultant dyspepsia, erosion, ulceration, haematemesis and melaena; slight blood loss may occur in about 70 per cent of patients with most aspirin preparations, whether buffered, soluble or plain, and often this is not accompanied by dyspepsia. Slight blood loss is not usually of clinical significance but may cause iron-deficiency anaemia during long-term salicylate therapy.

Incidentally, aspirin only began to be widely prescribed for arthritics when another 'wonder-drug' — cortisone — was found to have such dire effects on the metabolic and glandular functions of the patients that doctors turned to aspirin as a 'safer' alternative.

Laxatives have also been resorted to over the years in the belief that they could be taken safely and effectively for the relief of constipation. The same reference work from which we have already quoted comments that 'laxatives and the more drastic purgatives are commonly taken for constipation, but as this condition may result from a faulty diet lacking in vegetable fibre it is best treated initially by dietary adjustment'.

It goes on to warn that:

> ...the constant use of purgatives to induce a daily

habit, which is commonly believed to be necessary for good health, may decrease the sensitivity of the intestinal mucous membranes so that larger doses have to be taken and the bowel fails to respond to normal stimuli. Thus the redevelopment of a normal habit is prevented.

Unfortunately, no such warning is printed on the labels under which most of the proprietary laxatives are sold, and unless the sufferer is alerted to the dangers by an enlightened GP or a better-informed relative or friend the progressive deterioration in bowel function and tissue degeneration is inevitable.

Liquid paraffin is a laxative that was at one time widely used in the treatment of constipation because of its lubricant qualities and the fact that it softened the stools — a feature that recommended its use by patients suffering from haemorrhoids, fissure and other painful afflictions of the rectum and anus. Unfortunately, as some of these unfortunate patients found eventually, the laxative not only caused damage to the tissues of the intestines but also blocked the absorption into the bloodstream of the fat-soluble vitamins A and D. Prolonged dependence on the laxative was also reported to have caused pneumonia in apparently healthy individuals.

In view of what we have said in a preceding chapter concerning the important metabolic functions carried out by certain types of bacteria in a healthy colon, it is relevent to point out that the antibiotics such as penicillin, which have been prescribed so freely in the past, destroy both harmful and beneficial bacteria.

Following such treatment, therefore, it is necessary to restore normal bacterial balance in the digestive tract before the bowel can operate efficiently and carry out its proper assimilative functions.

The reader will be reminded of this necessary precaution when we explain the nature and purpose of the treatment measures which must be adopted in order to deal effectively with the various bowel disorders, the nature and symptoms of which we shall now explain.

7.

What's in a Name?

Bearing in mind the complexities of the digestive system and the wide variety of chemical processes with which it has to contend continuously throughout the seventy years or so which constitute the 'normal' life-span, it is not surprising that many things can and do go wrong from time to time.

No two human beings are the same either structurally or chemically, and each individual is endowed at birth with organic strengths and weaknesses. Most of us know people who claim to be able to 'eat anything' without showing the slightest sign of any digestive upset, while there are others who are plagued with recurring pains and other even more distressing symptoms despite the fact that they claim to exercise the greatest care in regard to their diet and other habits and activities.

In both cases, however, some degree of scepticism is justified, if only because the former individual may well be laying the foundations for the development of a gastric ulcer, or gallstones, or colitis, while the latter's avowed concern regarding diet, etc. may well be based on ignorance of basic nutritional principles as a result of which he or she is in fact subsisting on a totally inadequate or unbalanced diet.

When things do go wrong and a visit to the doctor's surgery becomes necessary, a name will be allotted to the patient's condition, depending on the nature and location of the symptoms, and subsequent treatment will be determined largely by the doctor's choice of a particular 'label' and with the primary objective of relieving the symptoms.

The nature cure approach is fundamentally different in that relatively little importance is attached to local symptoms. Instead, the main emphasis is placed on the need to relate them to the patient's diet and general life-style in order to determine what errors of omission or commission have been responsible for disrupting the system and what needs to be done to restore normal equilibrium.

Whereas someone suffering from colitis would expect his doctor to prescribe a different remedy from that provided for his neighbour who is afflicted with haemorrhoids, the naturopath may well find that both patients have come to grief from basically the same reasons, and so his advice to each of them will differ only in minor details. The logic that underlies this line of reasoning will, however, be more readily appreciated if we consider briefly the more common bowel troubles, explain what is meant by the 'labels' attached to them and the significance of their various symptoms.

Constipation and diarrhoea: There is no doubt

that constipation is a constant or recurring source of worry to many people. It is not, however, a 'disease' in the accepted sense of the term, nor does the word have the same meaning for all people.

Here again we come up against the recurring question, 'What is *normal*?' in the context of a bodily function. There is, of course, no simple or satisfactory answer, because there are so many variable factors which can change the body's rhythms and reactions quite dramatically from day to day and season to season.

As a very broad generalization it is probably reasonable to assume that the bowel will need to be emptied once in every twenty-four hours or so, but this interval may well be halved or doubled under certain circumstances without there being any cause for concern. The size of the meal, the nature of the foods of which it is comprised, the state of mind of the consumer, and any variation in the nature of his or her physical activities are but a few of the factors which may retard or accelerate the various digestive functions.

A diagnosis of constipation, therefore, is only justified when bowel function is slowed or suspended sufficiently to cause other symptoms. For example, the stools will have become hard and compacted due to the dehydration to which they are subjected during the protracted passage through the colon. Consequently, defecation will be difficult and perhaps painful, and the resultant rectal congestion may cause haemorrhoids and bleeding. The patient may feel lethargic, with poor appetite, headache, bad breath and coated tongue.

Such symptoms inevitably give rise to increasing apprehension and introspection in the sufferer, which, as explained in a previous chapter, will inhibit other digestive functions so that the problem becomes to some extent self-perpetuating.

If this state of affairs is allowed to persist the body's alarm signals are triggered off and emergency procedures are initiated in an effort to restore normal function. In response to the increasing distension and congestion in the bowel, the normal fluid extraction procedures are suspended and the irritated mucous membranes pour out a copious secretion of a clear, thin mucus similar to that which flows from the nostrils during a severe cold in the head. This fluid serves the dual purpose of liquefying the compacted faeces and lubricating the bowel walls, thus facilitating evacuation.

The same chain of events will be set in motion if tainted food or water or some other harmful substance has been ingested and which the body seeks to eliminate as quickly as possible. In this case the diarrhoea may be accompanied by violent vomiting so that the offending material is ejected before the processes of assimilation are set in motion, thus minimizing its harmful potential.

When the nature and causes of constipation and diarrhoea are understood it becomes clear why the use of laxatives and astringent drugs in the treatment of these two common bowel disorders is likely to be harmful rather than beneficial. Most of the former are irritants which goad an already weakened bowel to the point of exhaustion, while the use of the latter can only abort the body's efforts to clear the bowel of toxic substances.

Both methods of treatment, therefore, do no more than suppress the *symptoms* of functional disturbance, the causes of which are ignored. Inevitably, therefore, there is a progressive deterioration in the patient's condition and two relatively simple digestive disorders are complicated by degeneration of the maltreated intestinal tissues.

Appendicitis: The appendix is a long, thin, tubular appendage to the caecum (see Fig. 1, page 47) which is situated at the point where the small intestine empties into the colon. Physiologists have failed to identify any specific function that is performed by what they think may be a vestigial organ, but because it is composed partially of lymphatic tissue it is reasonable to assume that it contributes in some way to the body's defensive mechanisms.

The appendix is approximately 9cm ($3\frac{1}{2}$ in) in length and rather less than 1cm ($\frac{1}{3}$ in) in diameter, and because of its shape and situation it is understandably vulnerable to congestion and inflammation when the lower part of the colon becomes blocked and distended as a result of prolonged constipation. Food residues then ferment rapidly, and when faecal matter becomes trapped and immobilized in a narrow pocket of intestinal tissue it provides an ideal environment for the proliferation of harmful bacteria. It is a tribute to the effectiveness of the body's defence mechanisms that appendicitis is a relatively rare emergency, although during the first half of the twentieth century it became what, for want of a more suitable term, can only be described as a 'fashionable' diagnosis. As a result, many patients were rushed to hospital with abdominal pains and the surgeons were kept busy removing suspect appendices. Eventually, however, word began to seep through to the public that many of the organs thus removed were found to be either disease-free or only mildly inflamed, and enthusiasm for the operation gradually waned.

There are, of course, many possible causes of abdominal pain, but the symptoms of appendicitis are now well documented and fairly readily identifiable. Initially, there is acute pain near the navel in the centre of the abdomen which gradually moves down and to the right just above the groin. Prior to this, there will have been a history of constipation and perhaps sporadic diarrhoea, and the patient will feel generally out of sorts.

As the inflammation increases the pain will become even more severe and the patient will tend to lie on his or her back with the right leg drawn up in an effort to gain relief. There will be loss of appetite, as is invariably the case in all acute illnesses, and there will be some degree of feverishness. The muscles over the lower-right area of the abdomen will become tense and hard, and a slight swelling may become apparent within two or three days of the onset of the condition.

A first attack may clear spontaneously, but

unless proper treatment is initiated and the causes are removed it is likely that a more severe attack will occur later and surgical interference may then be unavoidable. In between these acute attacks there may be sporadic episodes of dull pain or discomfort in the affected area — a condition sometimes labelled 'grumbling appendix'. It constitutes a clear warning that serious trouble is simmering and that action needs to be taken as a matter of urgency to identify and remove the fundamental causes.

Acute appendicitis only manifests itself when the body's defence systems have been strained beyond endurance. By the time this stage has been reached inflammation can rapidly regress to ulceration or the formation of an abscess which may then perforate, releasing putrefying faecal matter into the abdominal cavity and causing generalized and possibly fatal peritonitis.

Mucous colitis — which is sometimes diagnosed as spastic colon — is a very debilitating condition which is most common in young or middle-aged women. It is characterized by persistent abdominal pain of a type not unlike that of appendicitis, but more frequently affecting the lower-left area, and usually most marked following a bowel movement.

Constipation is invariably a predisposing factor, with difficult passage of hard, ribbon-like stools, interspersed with bouts of diarrhoea during which copious amounts of stringy mucus may be passed, but no blood. There will be abdominal distension due to the constipation, and the fermentation of high-carbohydrate food residues will often give rise to bowel flatulence.

Colonic spasm is mainly an affliction of nervous individuals, which accords with what has been explained in a previous chapter in regard to the disrupting influence of worry and anxiety on the digestive sytem. Although overwork and mental or emotional stress are important contributory factors, attacks of this kind will only occur if the bowel has already been weakened as a result of faulty nutrition and other errors, including the habitual use of laxatives.

The characteristic pains and discomfort of this condition are triggered off by inflammation of the bowel lining which causes spasmodic cramp-like contractions of the muscle layers of the colon.

Ulcerative colitis: When the congestive and inflammatory bowel disorders have been allowed to persist or recur without any change in faulty feeding habits, while resorting to the use of laxative and other drugs to allay the symptoms, the condition of the mucous membranes which line the bowel will eventually degenerate to the point where they begin to disintegrate. When this occurs, ulcers will develop and blood will appear in the stools mixed with faeces and mucus. There will, of course, be the usual history of constipation and possibly of other digestive upsets with gastric discomfort, pain, hearturn, etc., for the relief of which the sufferer may have resorted to one of the proprietary antacid medicines.

Young adults are frequent victims of this

condition in which stress and worry are again an important contributory factor. As the congestion and ulceration permeate from the small intestine to the colon, attacks of diarrhoea become increasingly frequent and severe, as also do the accompanying griping pains. The debilitating effects of the blood-loss, impaired nutrition and the dehydration resulting from the recurring attacks of diarrhoea will take a heavy toll, resulting in progressive weight-loss and physical weakness.

Eventually, in the absence of conservative treatment, the condition will almost certainly become critical, and at this stage surgical intervention may be unavoidable, possibly involving the removal of part of the colon. This increasingly common operation — colostomy — necessitates forming an artificial outlet from the bowel through the abdominal wall through which the faeces are excreted into a disposable receptacle.

Haemorrhoids, or piles as they are frequently described, are a very common and painful affliction which is characterized by the development of varicose veins in the lining of the rectum. There are many possible causative factors including a faulty diet deficient in fibre, weak abdominal muscles due to lack of exercise, obesity and abdominal distension, tight belts, support garments and other constrictive items of clothing.

In short, all those factors which cause constipation will also predispose to piles by weakening and distending the abdomen, compressing the intestines and colon, and so restricting the circulation of blood from the lower limbs back to the heart. As a result, the veins in the pelvic basin become engorged and distended in exactly the same way as those in the calves and thighs become varicose. The problem is accentuated in the tissues of the rectum as a result of the physical pressure of hard, bulky faeces, and the sufferer's efforts to achieve a motion by straining at stool.

From time to time the engorged veins may rupture just inside the anus so that the faeces are stained with bright red blood. Defecation may be painful, and at times the discomfort may persist for a while after the passage of a stool. Irritation and inflammation of the anal tissues may also be troublesome in certain cases. These symptoms are often very distressing, but they seldom have serious health implications except in the more serious cases where the blood loss may aggravate anaemia.

Diverticular disease: A diverticulum is a small pouch of bowel-lining tissue which protrudes through the muscular wall of the colon in much the same way as a part of the small intestine pushes through the abdominal muscles to form a hernia. The condition was virtually unknown in Europe until late in the nineteenth century when refined sugar and white flour began to replace the coarser natural products in the conventional diet. The resulting absence of fibrous bulk in the faeces slowed down the digestive processes and impaired the peristaltic action of the intestines. This in turn caused distension of the colon and under the increasing internal pressure the weakened bowel walls eventually broke down and diverticulae were formed — a condition which is termed *diverticulosis*.

Initially, the condition may give rise to only mild discomfort and an occasional spasmodic abdominal pain resembling the symptoms already experienced by the sufferer as a result of the predisposing constipation and other mild digestive upsets. Usually, however, the diverticulae will proliferate and the trapped faecal matter will stagnate and cause inflammation and infection — a condition which is then termed *diverticulitis*. There is likely to be acute griping pain usually in the left side of the abdomen, with fever and sporadic attacks of diarrhoea.

In many cases it is only when these symptoms occur that the patient becomes sufficiently alarmed as to seek professional advice, and an X-ray examination readily confirms the diagnosis. At this stage, an abscess may form in the infected diverticulum and perforate into the abdominal cavity, causing peritonitis.

Cancer of the colon: Cancer constitutes the ultimate breakdown of the cellular structure of the body tissues as a result of long-sustained and intolerable chemical abuse and physical misuse. The tissues and fluids of which the human organism is constructed are believed to be made up of some two hundred different cells, the various components of which can only be derived from the food we eat, the liquids we drink and the air we breathe. When, as is increasingly common in industrialized communities, all of these elements are chemically manipulated and polluted it is inevitable that, sooner or later, the intricate and finely balanced processes employed by the body in the construction and maintenance of its many complex tissues will become hopelessly disorganized. As a result, 'rogue cells' will be formed which cannot be controlled and co-ordinated by the body's normal regulating mechanisms and which proliferate rapidly to form malignant tumours.

Because the colon is exposed to so much chemical and physical abuse it is a frequent site of malignancy, the early signs and symptoms of which are not unlike those of other bowel disorders such as ulcerative colitis, appendicitis and diverticulitis. Consequently, the true nature of the problem may not be identified until the tumour has enlarged to such an extent as to cause obstruction of the bowel, by which time the malignant cells may already have invaded the liver and other organs.

The disease processes will by then have passed the point of no return, and major surgery may do little more than delay the inevitable outcome by perhaps a few months or, at best, a year or two.

The reader cannot have failed to notice that throughout the preceding catalogue of bowel disorders a single common causative factor has been implicated — namely, constipation.

This needs to be borne in mind when, in the succeeding chapters, we go on to consider the natural treatment measures which need to be adopted in order to restore normal bowel function and provide the body with the materials which are needed to strengthen weakened and damaged tissues.

With the exception of ulcerative colitis and bowel cancer — the victims of which will almost certainly be under professional care — the problems with which we are concerned are all capable of resolution, given patience and perseverence, if sensible and logical steps are taken to correct the faulty dietetic and other habits which have weakened the body's innate capacity for repair and self-healing and caused the breakdown of a vital part of the digestive and assimilative system.

8.

The Logical Alternative

So far we have been concerned almost exclusively with the obstructive and destructive influences which insidiously — often over a period of many years or even decades — combine to wreak havoc with the functions and organs of the alimentary canal. This admittedly protracted preoccupation with so many varied negative forces is unavoidable if the reader is to be able to look back over his or her medical history and recognize what it is that he or she has done, or omitted to do, to bring about such dire consequences.

Only then will he or she be in a position to appreciate the rationale of the alternative, natural approach to these problems and be ready to embark on a course of reconstructive treatment with confidence and a clear understanding not only of *what* is required but — even more important — the reason *why* the various therapeutic measures are necessary for ultimate success.

To summarize, the fundamental tenet of

natural healing is that the human organism has an innate capacity for self-healing and self-repair which can achieve near miracles *provided that emcumbrances are removed and the necessary conditions and materials are provided*.

We are all well aware that, given warmth, rest and cleanliness, torn flesh will heal and broken bones will mend with little or no outside assistance. Surely, then, it is not difficult to accept the postulate that internal tissues and organs which have been misused and damaged will regenerate with equal facility if they are allowed to do so in their own time and without interference, no matter how well intended.

So what are the basic prerequisites for natural healing?

The first priority is to remove the obstructions from the bowel and thus relieve the internal pressure and congestion which are the direct cause of distension and inflammation. This essential prerequisite can only be achieved by discontinuing the input of unwanted food material — in other words, by undertaking a short period of therapeutic fasting. To the uninitiated, this may appear at first to be a drastic and rather daunting undertaking, but it should be remembered that a clogged digestive system is a very inefficient organ and that as a consequence only a small proportion of the food that is consumed will have been digested and assimilated. In a sense, therefore, the patient's body will already have been subjected to some degree of involuntary fasting, which is why such symptoms as fatigue, weight loss and nervous prostration are a feature of the type of bowel disorders with which we are concerned. Almost invariably, also, there is some degree of anorexia — loss of appetite — which is in fact a clear indication that the body wishes to be relieved of any further burden on the digestive system.

Unfortunately, civilized man has been conditioned from infancy onwards to believe that, no matter what his instinctive reactions may dictate, he *must* continue to eat in order to keep up his strength. So deeply is this conviction ingrained that even patients who are seriously ill in hospital will be cajoled into taking some form of liquid or solid food, even though the very sight or smell of it may evoke revulsion.

In this respect, wild and even domesticated animals will have no hesitation in obeying their natural instincts when the need arises. Faced with injury or illness, they will immediately stop eating, and no matter how much we may tempt them by offering their favourite delicacies they will steadfastly refuse to take anything except occasional drinks of water. They will tuck themselves away in a warm, dark corner and sleep or rest quietly until they are well on the way to recovery. Only then will these 'dumb' animals become gradually more active and begin to take food. Their instincts tell them what needs to be done in order that their innate self-healing processes may operate with maximum speed and efficacy, and nothing that we can do will divert them from the course they have set themselves.

By contrast, intelligent man allows himself to be persuaded by well-meaning but misguided relatives or medical advisers to ignore the clear directions provided by his natural instincts and 'feed to keep up his strength', take potentially harmful drugs which can only further deplete the vital resources of an already weakened system and meekly conform to the dictates of custom and tradition.

What should have been a tissue-cleansing and revitalizing procedure will have been frustrated, and inevitably the patient's condition will continue to deteriorate.

Although the 'three good meals a day' mentality is probably less widespread today than it was in the past, the daily ritual of eating at fixed mealtimes, regardless of bodily needs, is still observed by the vast majority of people in Western communities, and the prospect of missing even one meal will arouse some degree of apprehension. Therefore, the suggestion that anyone should voluntarily abstain from any kind of food for one, two or even three days will be met with incredulity and the prediction of the direst consequences.

It is a fact, however, that many millions of people throughout the world undertake such fasts regularly as part of their religious observances and consider themselves physically and mentally purified and uplifted as a consequence. And yet therapeutic fasting, which has always been regarded as probably the single most effective modality in the naturopathic armamentarium, is undoubtedly a very widely misunderstood and misrepresented procedure.

Much of the confusion has arisen because both the medical establishment and the press have tended to represent fasting as being synonymous with starvation, thus understandably instilling an element of fear in the minds of the public.

In order to allay this apprehension, the fundamental difference between therapeutic fasting and pathological starvation can be illustrated quite clearly by reference to the pictures of famine victims which, sadly, are all too frequently a familiar feature of television and press reports from Third-World countries. Here, the tragic effects of starvation are clearly apparent, particularly in the young children who are suffering and dying as a result of drought-induced crop failures. The sunken cheeks, emaciated arms and legs, staring eyes, distended and fluid-filled abdomens, protruding ribs and shoulder-blades and an air of apathy and hopelessness — these are the true and unmistakable signs of malnutrition which by no stretch of the imagination can possibly be compared with the effects of a short therapeutic fast conducted under carefully controlled conditions.

Very much longer fasts — up to forty days in some cases — have been employed by naturopaths in the treatment of serious chronic ailments, but in these cases the patients were under constant supervision in residential clinics.

With few exceptions, however, notably when a patient is already extremely weak and emaciated, nothing but good can come from a short fast conducted with reasonable care by a well-informed patient who has confidence in what he is doing and is not plagued by baseless doubts and fears. Not only will this simple exercise in self-discipline bring substantial health benefits but it will also impart a rewarding sense of achievement and mental satisfaction.

The short fast is undoubtedly the most efficient means of initiating the tissue-cleansing processes which are an essential preliminary to the constructive and restorative measures which will be employed once the bowel has been cleared of fermenting and damaging food residues. Faulty nutrition is certainly the major causative factor in constipation and the many more serious bowel disorders to which it gives rise, and all the time we continue to burden the alimentary system with unwanted food we are dissipating vital energy which is needed for the more important recuperative purposes.

Once the bowel has been cleared of debris, the next step is to cleanse its tissues and soothe the inflamed mucous membranes by means of a carefully restricted diet consisting solely of fresh fruit, and fruit and vegetable juices. The provision of highly alkaline elements, with a liberal vitamin content, in a basically fluid form but with an important fibrous element will have a soothing effect on the bowel linings, dilute and neutralize acid digestive secretions, and at the same time provide just sufficient bulk to encourage a gentle peristalsis and so facilitate the bowel cleansing processes.

In this way the digestive and eliminative organs are encouraged to return gradually to something approaching normal efficiency, so that they are able to take up essential nutrients and dispose of unwanted residues. The next stage, therefore, after having cleared the congested bowel, is to increase gradually the quantity and variety of wholesome but easily digested foods and so coax the digestive and eliminative organs into accepting a wider range of assimilative functions. This will be achieved by having frequent small meals of simple whole foods which are eaten slowly and masticated thoroughly, ensuring that the constituents are such as will produce a basically alkaline reaction when metabolized and absorbed into the blood-stream and other tissue fluids.

This means that for a further short period fruit and vegetables will predominate in the diet, ensuring, however, that they are cooked conservatively in order to retain essential nutrients and that salt and sugar are not added during the preparation.

Once this transitionary process has been completed, it wil be possible to amplify the diet still further and establish a properly balanced regime which will provide the body with all the essential nutrients which are needed to restore its tissues and organs to full functional efficiency.

At this stage it is timely to explain that what are sometimes termed 'acid fruits' do, in fact, have an alkaline reaction after being subjected to the chemical processes of digestion. It is the starches, sugars and animal proteins which are mainly responsible for what is commonly known as 'acid indigestion' or 'acidity', which is why naturopaths maintain that a properly balanced diet should consist of approximately 60 per cent of the alkaline fruits, vegetables and salads and not more than 20 per cent each of the acid-forming carbohydrates and proteins. Fats, in their pure, extracted form need have no place in such a diet, since the body's very limited needs in this respect will be met adequately by the fat content of other foods.

Such a regime will provide all the essential nutrients in their natural form and combinations, but we must stress once again the need for *quality* in our food while exercising moderation in regard to *quantity*.

We have mentioned that meat is one of the predominantly acid-forming foods and that fats need to be consumed only in the strictest moderation as part of a balanced diet, and so it is relevant at this stage to consider the reasons why many naturopaths advocate a lacto-vegetarian regime — i.e. one from which flesh foods are excluded and which relies instead on dairy produce, pulses, nuts, etc. to provide the protein component of the diet.

We will ignore the moral and humanitarian aspects of this very controversial subject which have aroused such widespread public concern and interest, and confine ourselves solely to considerations of health and nutrition.

The theory that meat is an essential component of the human diet has long since been abandoned by even the most conservative orthodox nutritionists, except perhaps those who have a vested commercial interest in the promotion of animal meat products, and there is no longer any reasonable doubt that lacto-vegetarian proteins are an adequate alternative.

Certainly, there are millions of healthy, well-nourished people throughout the world who totally exclude meat from their diet, and there are, in fact, strong anatomical and physiological facts which support the contention that man is not by nature a carnivore.

Naturopaths have long maintained that because of its acid properties and its liability to produce putrefactive residues in the alimentary tract, meat should have no place in the human diet. Our teeth, it is pointed out, are designed primarily to *grind* the food we eat, whereas those of the carnivores are long and pointed to enable them to tear flesh from the bones of their prey and swallow it with little or no premastication.

It is also pointed out that the chemical structure of the carnivore's digestive juices is very much more strongly acid than ours in order to facilitate the assimilation of flesh and bone, the residues of which are more rapidly excreted through a substantially shorter intestinal system than that with which man is equipped.

There is in fact increasing evidence to support the view that a diet containing a preponderance of meat and animal derivatives may be largely responsible for a number of serious organic diseases such as high blood-pressure, kidney failure and coronary heart disease, all of which have a high and increasing incidence in the prosperous, meat-eating Western communities. Moreover, these diseases which were once confined almost exclusively to the older age-groups are becoming increasingly rife among middle-aged and even younger people.

The latter fact highlights the importance of another aspect of the natural healing armamentarium which must be incorporated into any treatment programme which is designed to correct the functional disorders which are associated with colitis and other bowel troubles and facilitate the repair of damaged tissues — i.e. physical exercise.

We have already referred briefly to the part played by the blood and lymph circulatory systems in conveying nutrients to all the body's tissues and organs, removing waste products and neutralizing and destroying harmful bacteria and toxins. We have also explained the part which muscular activity plays in pumping the blood and lymph from the extremities back to the liver and heart for purification and reoxygenation. It will be appreciated, therefore, that the steady decline in the need for strenuous physical activity which has taken place throughout the twentieth century will have played a not inconsiderable part in predisposing the body to congestive and degenerative diseases, including constipation, colitis and haemorrhoids.

For decades now increasing reliance on the private car and public transport has virtually removed any need to use the legs for walking, and at the same time the ubiquitous television set has discouraged active participation in sports and physical recreational pursuits. Fortunately, it appears that a reaction is beginning to manifest itself and more and more people of all ages are finding an outlet for the long-suppressed instinctive desire for physical

expression. Rambling, jogging, squash,
swimming, fell-walking and the various team-
sports are all attracting new recruits, but many
middle-aged and older people are already
suffering the health penalties of earlier inertia,
including the bowel disorders with which we are
now concerned.

To repair the damage, therefore, it is essential
that the efficiency of the circulatory system
shall be restored by means of remedial exercises
aimed at strengthening the abdominal muscles,
combined with a progressive programme of
regular outdoor activity to stimulate the return
blood-flow through the abdomen.

For the former purpose we shall be explaining
a series of suitable exercises (see appendix A on
page 116) while to achieve the second objective
there is no better means than a daily brisk walk,
undertaken as a regular discipline and adjusted
in both duration and intensity with the aim of
achieving a gradual increase in physical capacity.

It is a simple physiological fact that the
strength and stamina of a muscle develop in
direct ratio to the demands that are made upon
it, hence the need for *regular* daily activity,
taking care, however, to avoid imposing undue
strain on weakened muscles in the early stages
of the treatment programme. The great value
of walking as a remedial exercise lies in the fact
that it involves virtually the entire muscular
system — arms, legs, abdomen, chest, buttocks
and shoulders, and when it is combined with
deep breathing the muscular diaphragm is
vigorously activated, rising and falling
rhythmically with each breath and so helping to

draw blood and lymph from the legs up through the pelvis and abdomen into the thoracic cavity and back to the heart. The latter organ, being composed of muscular tissue, benefits substantially from the increased work-load, becoming stronger and more efficient as a result and so better able to withstand the stresses and strains of daily life without incurring the risk of heart failure and coronary disease.

Older, retired people who are still physicaly active should have no difficulty in allocating the necessary time each day, and if a companion can be enlisted for company it is a good discipline to fix a set time and determine to venture forth regardless of the vagaries of the weather, other than really torrential rain, black ice or a blizzard! A pair of good walking boots or shoes will be found more comfortable than wellies, although the latter come into their own if there is mud, water or soft snow under foot. A lightweight and windproof anorak or similar hooded garment may be teamed with a pair of over-trousers such as those worn by golfers, skiers, ramblers, etc., and which can be purchased at quite reasonable cost from a sports outfitters.

Thus equipped, one is ready to venture out in most types of weather conditions and to return home with a physical glow and a satisfying sense of achievement.

Younger people who have occupational commitments and who use private or public transport to reach their office, shop or factory can, perhaps, adjust their timetables so that they can leave the car, bus or train a suitable distance from their destination and complete the journey on foot, reversing the procedure at the end of the day.

Housewives, too, may be able to follow a similar procedure when taking their children to school or when shopping or visiting friends. The children will share the benefits of the additional exercise.

A further bonus is achieved if, when walking, a conscious effort is made to straighten the spine, pulling in the abdomen and so helping to strengthen the muscles and gradually reduce any waistline distension.

Admittedly, all this necessitates the adjustment of established routines, but with a little patience and perseverance it will be found that the new habit-patterns can be incorporated into one's daily round without too much disruption and inconvenience, and with considerable benefit.

Having, therefore, defined the main priorities in regard to the natural approach to the various bowel disorders — i.e. the short fast, the adoption of a balanced and nutritious dietary regime, and an exercise routine designed to restore muscular and circulatory efficiency — we can now explain how these and a number of auxiliary measures will be incorporated into a detailed treatment programme.

9.

So Let's Clear the Decks ...

Because new ideas and concepts are often difficult to comprehend a certain amount of repetition and re-emphasis is, we feel, excusable, and indeed necessary, in order that the reader will be able and ready to put into practice a carefully co-ordinated sequence of therapeutic procedures. It is essential that he or she should know what each stage of the treament is meant to achieve and be able to understand the significance of any physical or functional reactions which may arise from time to time.

If, therefore, because of an understandable eagerness to get to grips with a worrying bowel problem, any reader has been tempted to skip the preceding chapters we would urge him or her not to be impatient and to go back to the beginning and do the essential groundwork which alone can ensure the desired results.

We have explained in the preceding chapter that the first and most important step along the road to recovery from the various bowel

disorders is a short period of total abstinence
from solid food, including gruels, soups, milk
and milk drinks, as well as stimulants such as
tea, coffee, cocoa and alcohol. The object is to
allow the digestive and assimilative systems to
rest completely so that all the body's energies
can be concentrated on the task of 'spring-
cleaning' the body tissues and fluids, and
eliminating unwanted and harmful residues
from the alimentary canal.

To this end, the commencement of the
treatment schedule should be carefully planned
so that for at least three or four days — and
preferably for a week or more — demands on
one's mental and physical resources are
minimized so that the maximum degree of rest
and relaxation can be assured. Here, again,
retired people should have little difficulty in
arranging their affairs with this end in mind,
particularly if the co-operation of a husband or
wife is forthcoming, but even those with family
or occupational commitments should endeavour
to arrange to have a weekend or a few days'
holiday so as to be reasonably free from their
more demanding responsibilities and able to rest
during the day, retire early, and ensure at least
eight hours of sound sleep.

These precautions are necessary because once
the tissue-cleansing processes get under way
they are likely to induce eliminative reactions
similar to those which characterize acute illness,
e.g. headache, cough, and a feeling of general
malaise. In some cases the symptoms may be
relatively mild, while others may react more
dramatically with a raised temperature,

increased mucus secretion, profuse perspiration, loss of appetite, sore throat, enlarged glands and coated tongue.

The onset of any such symptoms constitutes what is termed 'a healing crisis' and it is an indication that the body has begun the process of tissue-cleansing which we aim to encourage and facilitate. It is an indication also that no matter what maltreatment it may have been subjected to in the past, the body has still sufficient reserves of vital energy to mobilize its inner capacity for self-healing and self-preservation and put it to constructive use.

Unless this important point is clearly understood at this stage any such reaction which may occur during treatment may well be misunderstood and so give rise to unnecessary concern, especially if well-meaning relatives or friends predict dire consequences if one persists with these strange new treatment measures.

Such understandable forebodings can easily undermine confidence at a time when one is feeling somewhat under the weather. Far from being worried by these phenomena, one should be encouraged to weather the storm, such as it may be, confident in the knowledge that what appears to be a set-back is in fact a clear indication that vital self-healing reserves are already being brought into operation.

The first signs of the onset of such a healing crisis will usually become apparent within the first twenty-four hours of the commencement of the fast. The body's built-in time-clock will continue to demand food at the customary mealtimes, but if these demands are resisted and allayed by taking a drink of dilute fruit or vegetable juice the appetite will very quickly subside.

There is likely to be an increased desire for fluids to meet the body's need for additional liquid to serve as a solvent for the toxins which are being released into the blood-stream.

The eliminative activities will usually have peaked by the end of the third day, so the fast may be broken very gradually by taking small quantities of fresh fruit for a further two or three days and then increasing and varying the food intake progressively, taking care, however, to have only small meals of simple whole foods. At this stage it is advisable to avoid acid fruits such as oranges, grapefruit, lemons and rhubarb, choosing instead apples, pears, grapes, melon and an occasional ripe banana.

This regime will allow the digestive and assimilative systems to resume their normal functions, cleansed, refreshed and capable once more of taking up and utilizing the essential nutrients and eliminating unwanted residues.

It is understandable that after the first twenty-four hours or so the short-fast regime will have cut off the flow of chyme from the stomach into the intestines, thus reducing the stimulus which triggers the peristaltic contractions of the bowel. If the tissues are still somewhat inflamed or irritated, as is likely in colitis and diverticulitis, for example, the bowel may continue to function and there may even be some degree of looseness in the movements. In other cases, however, e.g. constipation and haemorrhoids, it may be necessary to use auxiliary measures to clear the colon. For this purpose the use of an enema provides a simple and effective solution to the problem if the necessary equipment is available.

What is known as a gravity douche is probably the most convenient and effective apparatus for self-administration. It consists of a rubber container, sometimes in the form of a hot-water bottle, to which one end of a length of rubber tubing is connected, with a nozzle and tap or clip at the other end. The bag, containing approximately 1 pint of lukewarm water, is suspended at a height of 4 or 5 feet and the patient kneels down with his back to it. The nozzle, lubricated with a little soap or petroleum jelly or olive oil, is inserted into the anus, then the patient bends forward with his chest close to the floor and by manipulating the tap or clip allows the water to flow into the rectum.

If griping or any other discomfort is experienced the flow should be slowed or stopped until it passes. When the container is empty the patient should remain in the same position for several minutes, kneading the abdomen gently with one hand, before removing the nozzle and emptying the bowel.

An alternative to the gravity douche is the bulb enema — a length of tubing with a rubber bulb in the centre which is squeezed to inject water from a bowl placed nearby on the floor.

Both of these appliances are sometimes obtainable from the surgical supplies department of the larger chemists or from a surgical supply store which may be located with the aid of the Yellow Pages telephone directory.

Failing this, however, a mild herbal laxative may be taken for a day or two at the conclusion of the fasting period, or a glass of one of the proprietary mineral waters, taken on rising and prior to retiring, may prove effective in some cases.

It should be clearly understood, however, that neither the enema nor the laxative should be resorted to unless constipation persists, because their routine use will tend to impede the restoration of normal bowel function.

To further encourage the latter there are two simple measures which should be adopted when going to the toilet, both of which help to provide the bowel with the natural nervous and physical stimulus of which we have been deprived by evolution and civilization.

There is no doubt that before the introduction of the modern water-closet defecation would have been effected by adopting a squatting position with the knees apart and the thighs fully flexed on to the abdomen. The latter would thus be braced and supported so as to enhance the contraction of the abdominal muscles and minimize strain, and at the same time the buttocks would be fully separated thus minimizing constriction in the anal region and possibly instigating the reflexes which induce the relaxation of the anal sphincters, the partial extrusion of the rectum and the muscular contractions which facilitate defecation.

All of these anatomical prerequisites are partially or totally obstructed when the modern high-seated water-closet is used, necessitating an unnatural sitting position which in turn inhibits the reflexes and muscular contractions, and so causes straining at stool.

Since we cannot lower the toilet seat, the only practicable way to overcome this problem is to provide a platform on which to raise the feet. In its simplest form this can be achieved by placing two blocks of wood approximately 25 cm (15 in) apart below the front rim of the pan, ensuring of course that they are large enough to be quite stable. Large books, such as children's annuals or old telephone directories, will serve the same purpose provided that they will take the weight of the body without sliding out of position.

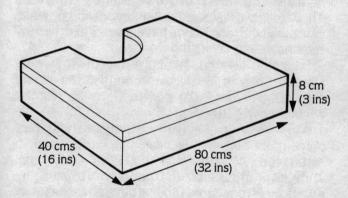

8 cm
(3 ins)

40 cms
(16 ins)

80 cms
(32 ins)

Figure 2   Toilet platform

If, however, the services of a handyman can be enlisted, a wooden platform similar to that illustrated in Fig. 2 can be constructed and used on a more or less permanent basis. The suggested measurements may be varied to some extent to meet individual needs, bearing in mind that the objective is to raise the knees and flex the thighs fully so that they brace and support the abdomen.

To further stimulate the nerve reflex which relaxes the anal sphincters and facilitates the peristaltic contractions of the rectum the hands should be placed behind the back, so that the fingertips are touching just above the anus and, pressing gently but firmly, the fingers should be pulled upwards and outwards, maintaining the pressure for a few seconds while contracting and pressing down with the abdominal muscles. Then, after relaxing for a short while, the sequence is repeated rhythmically for up to ten minutes or until a bowel movement is achieved. This 'toilet drill' should be practised at least twice daily, preferably on rising and just before retiring.

Straining at stool should be avoided, relying instead on a gradual restoration of the nerve reflexes and muscular contractions to restore normal bowel function.

As we have explained in a previous chapter, steps must be taken to deal with weakness and distension of the abdominal muscles and stimulate circulation in the pelvic organs. In addition to regular outdoor exercise, this entails practising at least once daily the planned sequence of remedial exercises which are described and illustrated in Appendix A on page 116.

It is emphasized that discretion is necessary in the early stages of treatment to guard against over-enthusiasm and the possibility of straining and damaging weakened muscles and supporting tissues. The aim should be to keep comfortably within one's physical limitations and relax for a short time between movements so as to build up gradually the strength and endurance of the abdominal muscles.

Care needs to be taken also in the choice of clothing in order to avoid constriction around the waist and thighs which may impede the circulation of blood and lymph and so cause congestion in the lower limbs and pelvis. Tight belts, suspenders, waistbands and support garments should be dispensed with whenever possible, and the clothing generally should be as light and well ventilated as circumstances permit.

Having digressed from outlining a co-ordinated treatment programme in order to explain the auxiliary procedures which must be carried out in conjunction with the main therapeutic regime, we can now return to the latter.

We have completed the short fast and begun taking light meals of fruit in order to continue the tissue-cleansing and soothe the congested bowel lining. At this stage it is important that the beneficial bacteria which inhabit the healthy bowel are recolonized, since they are likely to have been depleted, or even destroyed, as a result of the abnormal disease conditions and the taking of laxatives and drugs, particularly the antibiotics.

By far the most efficient means of achieving this objective is to include natural, unflavoured yogurt in the diet at the earliest possible moment, and so a carton of this product will be added to the fruit meals once the fast is broken.

In addition to its beneficial effect on the bowel bacteria, yogurt provides a small but easily digested amount of protein and calcium and it also has a mild laxative effect to supplement that of the fruit fibre. Care must be taken, however, to avoid the artificially coloured and flavoured commercial yogurts.

With the completion of the fast and the cleansing diet, the first and most demanding phase of the treatment plan will have been completed. Our next objective is to progress to a dietary regime composed of natural, unspoilt foods which contain all the essential nutrients in the balanced proportions necessary to facilitate tissue repair and restore functional efficiency.

Initially, the emphasis will be on small meals of conservatively cooked vegetables with an egg or cheese dish and small quantities of raw and cooked fruit or soaked or stewed dried fruit, complemented by a little cereal food in the form of a slice or two of wholemeal bread or toast, brown rice, or muesli.

Meals of this kind, besides being very nutritious, are easily digested and contain just sufficient natural fibre to coax the weakened digestive tract to resume gentle peristaltic contractions without strain. Too often, nowadays, sufferers from bowel disorders are told that salvation lies in having a high-fibre diet and they may even be advised merely to take quite large quantities of bran in addition to their ordinary meals.

In the light of what has been explained in the preceding chapters it is not difficult to appreciate why the unfortunate patient's condition continues to worsen after the bowel has been whipped briefly into activity by the sudden surge of bulky and irritant fibre. A tired and weakened bowel needs to be soothed and coaxed gently back to functional normality after perhaps suffering years of maltreatment, and patience and perseverence are called for if a lasting solution is to be found to these distressing problems.

The patient's mental attitude may be just as much in need of adjustment as his dietary and physical habits, bearing in mind the effect of stress and anxiety on the digestive system. That is why, in the early stages of treatment at least, it is essential to rest and relax as much as possible and to retire early so as to ensure at least eight hours of sound sleep.

Although for this purpose the bedroom should be darkened and insulated from outside noise as far as possible, good ventilation is also essential to ensure that oxygen-depletion does not occur during the night. If, therefore, a window cannot be left ajar, the bedroom door should remain at least partially open.

If sleep does not come readily, it is a mistake to get up or switch on the light and read, since these practices merely stimulate the senses and make subsequent attempts to sleep more difficult. Instead, a comfortable position should be taken, with the eyes closed, and the neck, arms, legs, etc. should be allowed to relax as fully as possible. Mental relaxation will be encouraged if the thoughts are concentrated — for want of a more appropriate word — on memories of a pleasant holiday scene, such as lying on a beach in the sun, listening to the sounds of the waves, gulls, etc. This ensures that disturbing thoughts and anxieties are excluded, since the mind can follow only one train of thought at a time.

Having now reviewed at some length the various natural therapeutic measures which, in the following pages, we shall incorporate into a comprehensive, day-to-day treatment schedule, we would once again urge the reader to re-read the preceding pages if it is felt necessary to ensure familiarity with what he or she will be required to do as a preliminary to embarking on the road to recovery.

Sufferers from bowel disorders will be heartened to know that the cells which form the lining of the healthy intestines are sloughed off and renewed more rapidly than those of any other organ — usually within forty-eight hours or so. Clearly, it would be over-optimistic to expect diseased or damaged tissues to be rebuilt with the same facility, but knowledge of this phenomenon should encourage the reader to make the necessary effort to gradually restore the body's innate capacity for self-healing.

Those who have suffered only sporadic bouts of constipation, diarrhoea, flatulence or haemorrhoids may expect progressive improvement over a period of two or three months, but in cases of chronic disorders such as mucous colitis, 'irritable bowel', diverticulitis and 'grumbling appendix' the suggested treatment may have to be repeated at intervals of two or three months until normal bowel function is restored.

10.

... and Head for Health!

Now we are ready to assemble the various treatment measures which we have discussed in the preceding chapters and set them out to comprise a daily schedule covering a period of three weeks. At the conclusion the bowel should have been spring-cleaned of any overload of food residues, while inflamed mucous linings will have been soothed and encouraged to function more efficiently by the alkalizing diet.

We shall then suggest a week's menus to exemplify the type of wholefood diet which needs to be adopted in order that functional improvements may be consolidated and the self-healing processes may continue to restore damaged tissues and organs.

It is appreciated that in some cases domestic and business commitments may make it necessary to vary the time sequence of some elements of the programme, and discretion may be exercised in this respect provided that the daily dietary instructions are complied with conscientiously. For example, it is permissible to transpose the meals, but not to change the components, and the exercise sessions may be fitted into the daily routine at the most convenient times.

Before embarking on the treatment course, it remains only to offer a few final precautionary notes:

1. Tap water should be boiled for drinking purposes to remove chlorine, but bottled mineral water is preferable until normal bowel function is restored.

2. Hot baths are weakening and cause circulatory congestion so that the body becomes more susceptible to chilling. Cool or cold baths, on the other hand, are stimulating and they strengthen the blood-vessels. Take the former if necessary to promote relaxation just before retiring, but have a cool or cold sponge-down or shower on rising, followed by a brisk friction-rub with a skin-brush or very coarse towel.

3. Very hot foods and drinks can harm the delicate tissues of the alimentary canal and inhibit the secretion of digestive juices.

4. Have one-course meals only, eat slowly and masticate thoroughly. Avoid complex mixtures.

5. A little celery salt may be added when cooking vegetables if desired, but houshold salt, pepper, curry and other condiments and seasonings should not be used.

6. Sugar and synthetic sweeteners must not

be used. A little honey may be added to drinks, stewed fruits, etc. if desired.

7. Do not worry if there is some initial weight loss. Normal weight will be restored as a result of improved digestion and assimilation.

8. Any abdominal discomfort or pain that is experienced can be relieved by the application of a hot compress. Wring out a piece of cotton material, e.g. old sheeting, in hot water, fold into several thicknesses, apply to the abdomen and cover with a thick dry towel to retain the heat. Retire to bed with a hot-water bottle at the feet. Re-heat as necessary, and wash or replace the compress material the following day.

9. At all times, consciously maintain good posture with the spine straight, the knees braced when standing and the abdominal muscles contracted. Avoid slumping and stooping which restrict breathing and weaken and distend the abdomen.

10. Drinks should be taken as necessary to allay thirst. Fruit and vegetable juices should be mixed with an equal quantity of water. They are best made freshly when needed with the aid of an electric juice extractor or a hand-operated juice press. Alternatively, unsweetened canned or bottled juices may be purchased from health-food stores or some chemists or general stores.

11. Slippery elm food — also obtainable from health-food stores and some chemists — has a soothing effect on inflamed mucous

membranes. It also encourages peristalsis and, taken as a nightcap, promotes sound sleep.

With these injunctions in mind we are now ready to take the first steps which will help to bring relief and provide the only effective safeguard against the other organic and systemic disorders which plague so many people today.

1st DAY

1. *On rising:* Toilet drill (see page 100).
2. Glass of water or diluted juice sipped slowly. No solid food or other liquids *of any kind* may be taken throughout the day.
3. Cool or cold sponge-down followed by friction-rub.
4. Abdominal exercises (see Appendix A, page 116).
5. Outdoor exercise if possible, e.g. half-hour walk combined with deep-breathing. In hot weather have sponge-down and friction-rub on return and change clothing if necessary.
6. Drink of water or juice if needed.
7. Rest and relax for half hour or more if possible.
8. Normal activities as necessary during the day, but avoid as far as possible those involving undue mental or physical strain. Take drinks as needed and rest from time to time, preferably lying down in a darkened room.

9. *Early evening:* Outdoor exercise if practicable and drinks as needed.
10. *Before retiring:* Abdominal exercises followed by moderately hot bath if desired to promote relaxation. Retire early in a darkened but ventilated bedroom.

2nd and 3rd DAYS

Repeat first day's schedule, but if feeling tired or experiencing headache or other 'healing crisis' symptoms dispense with sponge-down and outdoor exercise. Have as much rest as possible, preferably in a darkened room.

Use the enema (see page 97) on third day if there has been no bowel movement.

4th DAY

1. *On rising:* Toilet drill.
2. Glass of water or juice.
3. Sponge-down and friction-rub.
4. Abdominal exercises.
5. *Breakfast:* Dish of stewed apple or prunes with 140ml ($\frac{1}{4}$ pt) unflavoured yogurt.
6. Outdoor exercise if desired, followed by sponge-down and friction-rub.
7. Drinks of water or juice as needed between meals.
8. *Midday:* As for breakfast or, if preferred, an apple, a pear and a few grapes (remove pips).
9. Normal activities as necessary, interspersed with rest periods when possible.
10. *Early evening:* As midday meal. Outdoor exercise, if desired, followed by sponge-down and friction-rub, preferably before

the meal or not less than one hour afterwards.

11. *Before retiring:* Abdominal exercises followed by moderately hot bath if desired.

Toilet drill, and enema if necessary.

Cup of slippery elm food mixed thinly with warm water and sweetened if necessary with a teaspoon of honey.

5th and 6th DAYS
Repeat fourth day's schedule, but ensure that outdoor exercise is taken at least once during the day, preferably before the evening meal or not less than one hour afterwards.

If constipated, use the enema or herbal laxative, provided that it has not been needed on either of the two previous days.

7th and 8th DAYS
Adapt the following daily programme as necessary to fit in with normal commitments.

1. *On rising:* Toilet drill.
2. Glass of water or juice.
3. Sponge-down and friction-rub.
4. Abdominal exercises.
5. *Breakfast:* Fruit and yogurt as on preceding days.
6. Outdoor exercise if possible followed by sponge-down and friction-rub.
7. Drinks of water or juice as needed.
8. *Midday:* Fruit and yogurt as on preceding days, but include a ripe banana.

9. Outdoor exercise, sponge-down and friction-rub.
10. *Evening meal:* Small serving of two conservatively cooked vegetables (choose from carrot, cabbage, sprouts, parsnip, broccoli, leek and onion, but not potatoes), with a scrambled egg or one tablespoon of cottage cheese.
11. *Before retiring:* Abdominal exercises. Toilet drill. Cup of slippery elm food.

9th and 10th DAYS
As for preceding days *except:*

1. *Evening meal:* A conservatively cooked or baked jacket potato may be taken with one green and one root vegetable, with a poached or scrambled egg, or a small omelette, or cream cheese, or sprinkled with 30 g (1 oz) grated nuts — e.g. hazels, walnuts, almonds, peanuts, etc.
Use the enema or laxative only if there has been no bowel movement for forty-eight hours.

11th to 14th DAYS
As preceding days except:

1. *Midday:* Small mixed salad of lettuce or grated cabbage, watercress, tomato, grated raw carrot, 30g (1 oz) washed raisins or sultanas, sprinkled with 30g (1 oz) grated nuts or 60g (2 oz) grated cheese. Eat slowly and masticate thoroughly. If any digestive discomfort is experienced revert to fruit and yogurt.

2. A moderately hot bath may be taken *once weekly* before retiring, or in the morning if preferred. In the latter case it should be followed by the sponge-down and friction-rub.

3. The enema or laxative should no longer be necessary, but may be used at intervals of four or five days if the bowel continues to be sluggish. Aim to dispense with either recourse as soon as possible.

15th DAY ONWARDS

1. *On rising:* Toilet drill.
2. Glass of water or juice.
3. Sponge-down and friction-rub.
4. Abdominal exercises if convenient.
5. *Breakfast:* See menus in Appendix B, page 121.
6. Drinks as needed between meals. Not more than two cups of weak unsweetened tea or decaffeinated coffee may be taken during the day if desired in place of the usual drinks.
7. *Midday:* See menus in Appendix B, page 121.
8. Outdoor exercise should be taken at any time(s) during the day when convenient, extending to a total of one hour's duration if possible, and followed by the sponge-down and friction-rub.
9. *Evening meal:* See menus in Appendix B on page 121.
10. *Before retiring:* Abdominal exercises. Cup of slippery elm food if desired.

11.

Keep Going!

As we have stressed in the preceding pages, the bowel disorders with which we are concerned have not been 'caught' overnight. They are the result of a process of atrophy and degeneration which, for many years perhaps, has disorganized the chemical processes of the digestive system and weakened and eroded its tissues.

Inevitably, therefore, time will be needed to restore metabolic equilibrium and repair the damage that has been wrought. The rate of progress towards recovery will be governed by many factors, including the nature, duration and severity of the bowel disorder and the age, previous health history and present physical and nervous resources of the patient.

Nevertheless, after taking account of all these variables, the overriding factors which ultimately will determine the rate of recovery will be the patient's own determination and willingness to achieve salvation *by his or her own efforts*, instead of relying misguidedly on the easy option of the pill and medicine bottle.

The incentive which is offered to those who

are prepared to make short-term sacrifices and change long-established habits is not merely the prospect of freedom from the pain, inconvenience and embarrassment of disordered bowel function. There is the inestimable bonus that, in solving the *specific* health problem, the structural and functional integrity of *the whole body* will have been strengthened, thus restoring the natural defence mechanisms which alone can afford a high degree of immunity to both acute and chronic illness.

Man is undoubtedly a creature of habit, but given the necessary incentive, coupled with patience and perseverance, even the most deeply entrenched habits can be changed. Once the new patterns are established, however, it is possible to look back with a deep sense of satisfaction at having, by one's own efforts, solved a complex problem and earned the priceless reward of lasting health.

The treatment schedule set out in the preceding pages will have released, or rather reactivated, the body's innate powers of self-healing. On completion of the initial programme, the simple health-promoting regime laid down for Day 15 onwards will consolidate the restorative processes which have been set in motion.

The specimen menus are, of course, meant only to serve as a guide to the type of meals and food combinations which, for many people, will sustain health and physical fitness, but there is ample scope for variation with regard to the wholefood dishes which may be substituted for the main meals which we have specified provided that the basic principles of healthful feeding are borne in mind: choose *whole* foods whenever possible; do not over-eat; do not have a large meal when very tired or worried; eat slowly; masticate thoroughly.

If help is needed in the selection of a healthful diet, a wide range of excellent wholefood cookery books is available from the publishers of this book, and a selection is usually to be found on the shelves of health-food stores and good bookshops.

Finally, we would remind readers that, in some cases, what appear to be temporary setbacks may occur from time to time during the early stages of treatment, in the form of sporadic bouts of constipation and/or diarrhoea, flatulence or abdominal discomfort. Any such eventuality is the cue for a reversion to the initial cleansing programme, but even in the absence of any such contingency it is advisable to undertake a second or even a third course of treatment at intervals of two or three months until all signs and symptoms of bowel weakness have been eliminated.

We cannot stress too strongly or too often that the rewards in terms of lasting health are strictly in accordance with, and proportional to, one's own efforts and determination, based on knowledge and understanding.

There can be no higher or more rewarding achievement than the restoration of good health, fitness and vitality.

Appendix A

Abdominal Exercises

These exercises are designed to strengthen the muscles of the abdomen and reduce distension. For the maximum benefit they should be practised twice daily — on rising and during the evening, but not less than one hour after a meal.

If at first any movement proves to be beyond one's physical capacity it should be omitted from the programme for a time, concentrating instead on the less demanding movements.

The aim should be to *develop the muscles progressively* by gradually increasing the range of movement and the number of repetitions, taking care to avoid undue strain. Initially, one or two repetitions of each movement may be all that can be achieved, but over a period of several weeks it should be possible to manage between ten and twenty repetitions, depending upon the nature of the exercise and the patient's innate physical resources.

1. Lie on the back with the hands resting on the lower abdomen and raise the legs slowly, keeping the knees straight, until the feet are clear of the floor, then lower and relax. The abdominal muscles will be felt to contract and harden as the legs are raised and then relax and soften when they are lowered. As the abdomen becomes stronger, the legs can be held in the raised position for a few seconds before returning to the starting position.

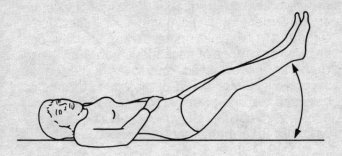

2. From the same starting position but with the arms splayed and the hands pressing on the floor, raise the legs to the vertical position with the knees straight, then separate them as widely as possible and close again, pressing the knees and ankles together strongly, repeating three or four times before lowering the legs and relaxing.

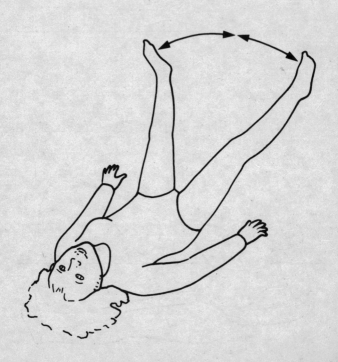

3. Lie on the back with the feet anchored and the hands resting on the lower abdomen, then rise slowly to a sitting position, return to starting position and relax.

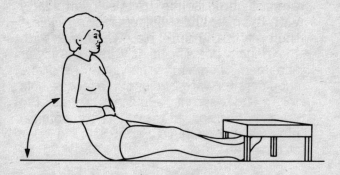

4. From the same starting position, raise the head and shoulders clear of the floor and rotate them first to the right, then to the left, and then return to starting position and relax.

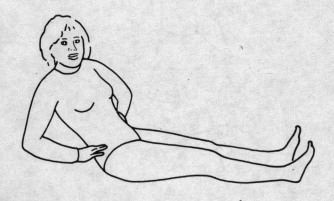

5. The following exercise can be practised conveniently and unobtrusively at any time when seated in an armchair or on a settee, and so it serves as a useful auxiliary means of consolidating the benefits of the main exercise programme. Settle comfortably with the head and shoulders resting against the back of the chair, place the hands with the fingers pressing gently into the lower abdomen, then simply move the head and shoulders forward two or three inches, hold for a few seconds, and return to the starting position and relax. The abdominal muscles will be felt to contract and relax alternately.

Appendix B

A Week's Menus...

The following menus are illustrative of the type of balanced meals which will satisfy most 'normal' appetites. Some discretion may, however, be exercised in regard to the choice of foods, the amounts served and the timing of the meals, provided that the overall balance conforms approximately with the 60:20:20 ratios explained on page 26.

Non-vegetarians may substitute 80 or 90g (3 oz) of meat, fish or poultry for the protein part of the meal if desired, but fried and fatty foods should be avoided.

If wholewheat bread causes indigestion or flatulence initially it is permissible to substitute one of the lower extraction loaves, i.e. those described as 'brown', 'farmhouse', 'granary', etc., for a time before gradually reverting to 100 per cent wholewheat bread as tolerance is established.

Any vegetables, fruits or salads which are not in season may be replaced by similar items.

Fruit should always be fully ripe. Sour or unripe fruit should never be eaten even when cooked.

Proprietary 'salad creams', dressings, sauces, table salt and other condiments should never be served. A little celery salt may be submitted if desired. Salad may be dressed with a little yogurt or no more than a dessertspoonful of olive or corn oil mixed with a teaspoonful of fresh lemon or orange juice.

1st DAY

Breakfast: Soaked or stewed dried fruit with yogurt.

Midday: Scrambled egg on two slices of wholewheat toast. An apple and a banana.

Evening: Cauliflower cheese with two medium potatoes and carrots or peas.

2nd DAY

Breakfast: Muesli (see recipe on page 124).

Midday: Lettuce and chopped celery with cottage cheese, sprinkled with washed raisins or sultanas.

Evening: Millet savoury (see recipe on page 125) with steamed cabbage and carrots.

3rd DAY

Breakfast: Stewed prunes with yogurt.

Midday: Three slices of wholewheat bread spread with mashed banana and washed sultanas.

Evening: Wholewheat spaghetti with two medium potatoes and one root and one green vegetable, conservatively cooked.

4th DAY

Breakfast: Poached egg on two slices of wholewheat toast.

Midday: Small salad of lettuce, tomato, grated carrot, etc. sprinkled with 30g (1 oz) grated nuts or 60g (2 oz) grated cheese.

Evening: Lentil roast (see recipe on page 125) with baked jacket potato and a green vegetable.

5th DAY

Breakfast: Muesli.

Midday: Two or three slices of wholewheat bread or crispbread with cream cheese and an apple or pear.

Evening: Mixed salad (see recipe on page 126.

6th DAY

Breakfast: Half grapefruit sweetened if necessary with a little melted honey and 140ml ($\frac{1}{4}$ pint) natural yogurt with sliced banana.

Midday: Stewed apple with chopped dates or raisins and yogurt.

Evening: Plain omelette with peas and potatoes (washed thoroughly and cooked in their skins).

7th DAY

Breakfast: Any fresh fruit, e.g. apple, pear, grapes, banana, etc., or stewed prunes or other dried fruit with yogurt.

Midday: Small salad of lettuce, tomato, celery, etc. with sliced banana and yogurt.

Evening: Mixed vegetable casserole sprinkled with 60g (2 oz) grated cheese.

RECIPES

Muesli

Ready-mixed muesli-base may be purchased from health-food stores, but coarse oatmeal is an economical alternative to provide a very nutritious and satisfying breakfast dish or a light midday or evening meal.

Ingredients: 2 or 3 heaped tablespoonsful muesli-base or coarse oatmeal
1 level dessertspoonful honey (optional)
1 heaped dessertspoonful washed raisins, sultanas or chopped dates
2 heaped dessertspoonsful nuts (hazels, peanuts, almonds, etc.)
$\frac{1}{2}$ medium apple
$\frac{1}{2}$ ripe banana
4 dessertspoonsful warm water

Mix the dried fruit into the cereal, melt the honey (if desired) into the warm water, pour over the cereal and leave to soak for one hour or overnight. Before serving, add grated apple, sprinkle over the grated nuts and decorate with banana slices.

Lentil Roast

Ingredients: 450g (1 lb) lentils
1 large onion
2 medium potatoes
Wholemeal breadcrumbs
Mixed herbs

Wash the lentils and boil until soft, then strain and mash and mix in the chopped onion and the potatoes (also boiled and mashed), adding the mixed herbs to taste.

Add breadcrumbs (if necessary) until the mixture is firm, then form into a roll, place in an oiled tin and bake until brown (approximately 30 minutes).

Millet Savoury

Ingredients: 2 tablespoons millet
3 medium tomatoes
1 clove garlic
1 level teaspoon yeast extract (Marmite, Vecon, etc.)
275ml ($\frac{1}{2}$ pt) water

Put the skinned and sliced tomatoes in a pan with the crushed garlic, pour over the water, stir in the yeast extract and bring to the boil. Add the millet, stir well, then cover and simmer until the water is absorbed (approximately 15 minutes).

When sufficiently dry, sprinkle with chopped parsley and serve.

Mixed Salad

A good, mixed salad is a meal in the true sense of the word, and it has the added merit that it can be prepared and cleared more quickly than many cooked meals.

The following combination will serve as a base which is capable of almost infinite variations according to taste and availability of the ingredients.

It can be further supplemented by one or two slices of wholewheat toast or crispbread spread thinly with yeast extract, peanut butter or honey.

Ingredients: Lettuce, tomato, beetroot (raw or cooked — no vinegar), celery, cucumber
1 dessertspoonful washed dried fruit — e.g. raisins, sultanas, dates, etc.
2 dessertspoonsful nuts — e.g. peanuts, cashews, almonds, hazels, etc.
60g (2 oz) cheese
½ medium apple
½ medium banana

Tear the lettuce leaves into pieces and line a large plate, then decorate with sliced tomato, cucumber, celery and grated or sliced beetroot.

Dice the apple into small pieces and scatter over, followed by the dried fruit, and finally grate the cheese and scatter over, followed by the grated nuts, and decorate with sliced banana.

Index